MAMA DRAMA

A Journey with Bipolar and
Dementia—Finding Light Through
Loss and Grief

SHERI SMITH

MAMA DRAMA
A Journey with Bipolar and Dementia—
Finding Light Through Loss and Grief

ISBN: 979-8-9923166-4-3 (Hardcover)
ISBN: 979-8-9923166-5-0 (Paperback)
ISBN: 979-8-9923166-6-7 (Audiobook)
ISBN: 979-8-9923166-7-4 (Ebook)

Disclaimer: This story was inspired by true events. To respect the privacy of individuals and maintain the integrity of the narrative, names, identifying details, and certain events in this book have been altered or fictionalized. Any resemblance to actual persons, living or deceased, is entirely coincidental.

Book Cover Design and Interior Formatting by 100Covers.

For my Mama, whose life and struggles form the heart of this book, and my fur son Ray, my beloved Rayla. You both are woven into every page. And all my beloved people and animals who have passed on, guiding me along this journey and keeping me inspired as I wrote.

Table of Contents

Foreword

By Pauline Parry, Author of My Culinary Love Story

It was nearly three decades ago that Sheri Smith came into my life. I was teaching at an event industry conference in Las Vegas and noticed a woman in the audience whose wide-open eyes hung on every word I said. I smiled to myself, thinking she might rush the stage after my presentation, but instead, I watched her quietly walk out of the room. Before she left, she turned around, our eyes met, and then she was gone.

It sounds like the beginning of a love story, and in many ways, it was. That evening, our paths crossed again, and this time she stopped to introduce herself. From that moment, our friendship began. Sheri, I believe, is one of a kind—a New Yorker who bubbles with excitement, often on the loud side, but only when she's comfortable with the people around her. Otherwise, she has a quiet, demure shyness about her. She has strong opinions and a hard edge, as she is quite cautious about who she lets into her life. Over the years, I've come to admire this about her, as it reflects her strength and self-preservation.

And why wouldn't she be careful? Her life has been marked by profound challenges—the struggles of living with her husband's bipolar and her mother's dementia, betrayal by her family, the loss of the castle she built on the Big Island that took ten years, and the devastating grief of losing her "heart" dog, Ray. These events turned her world upside down, forcing her to confront immense pain and emotional turmoil.

This book is raw and heartfelt, with glimmers of humor that have undoubtedly helped Sheri through her toughest moments. Her ability to adapt, find strength, and forgive shines through as she navigates and explores life with the support of friendship, community, and spirituality.

You will be inspired by how Sheri not only survived the complexities of her life but also took control of her circumstances to create a better future for herself. Her journey demonstrates incredible tenacity and resilience. Many of you will find her story relatable and may even draw strength from her experiences.

Sheri has shown me what true friendship is—a bond that endures through thick and thin. I am proud that she is sharing her life story with the world, as it will provoke thought, inspire determination, and remind readers that even in the face of adversity, it is possible to emerge stronger.

With love, Pauline Parry

Preface

This story explores the impact of heart-wrenching loss and betrayal. It delves into the depths of profound grief, illuminating the roles we're sometimes thrust into, ready or not. Through this journey, one can witness the resilience of the human spirit in the face of life's cruelest turns. I hope it serves as a poignant reminder of the capacity to endure, even when the weight of responsibility and sorrow threatens to break us.

I was "mama" to my German Shepherd, Ray. From a young age, I knew I would never have children—I always said I loved animals more than humans. Ray wasn't just a dog; he was my soulmate, my heart dog. It's a "thing"—a once-in-a-lifetime bond that can alter your life in all the best ways. He filled my life with the kind of love that only those who've experienced such a bond can understand. In 2014, at only seven years of age, as his health declined, I was forced to make the agonizing decision to "do my duty" and put him down. His loss shattered me and led me into prolonged grief disorder, something I hadn't known existed until I found myself living it.

I didn't get to care for my Mama as she descended into the depths of dementia since my cousin deprived me of the final years I could have had with her by hiding her whereabouts. My inheritance (the money) didn't matter since that was dust (can't take it with you). He took her and took control of her life and hid her from me. This writing is not just a personal story—it's a cautionary tale about family. The people you hope will help and support you can sometimes turn into your greatest opponents or adversaries. My cousin's actions revealed a cruelty and greed that I still struggle to comprehend.

Long before Ray, my ex-husband, J (a name I can't bear to say or write), became my first unexpected caregiving challenge. He struggled with undiagnosed bipolar disorder. No one spoke about these things back then. Thank the Lord this has changed! Nonetheless, I found myself taking on a role I never wanted: being a "mama" to a grown man who couldn't manage the basic tasks of life without constant help or reminders. The mental illness brought chaos into our home, and it reshaped the way I understood love, care, and responsibility. Untreated bipolar wreaked havoc on both our lives for twenty years. Twenty years of hell, abuse and bullying. Although I'm sure if you asked him today about those years he would beg to differ.

While all of this was happening, I was sustained by the memory and love of my fathers,

Nat and George. Nat allowed George to adopt me so I could be his heir and beneficiary. Nat, my bio dad, passed from cancer in 1973, and George, my "adopted" father, passed in the 90s. I was blessed to have two fathers who loved me so deeply.

I have always said after any event in my life (good or bad), "What am I meant to learn?" And my next thought was always, "What am I meant to share?" Oprah says, "Everyone has a story." This is mine—one of love (aloha), loss, betrayal, resilience, and the unexpected roles life forces us into when we least expect it.

For updates and future releases: Buy Now or Follow the Author

Website | Instagram | Facebook | LinkedIn | YouTube

Growing up in the '50s and '60s

My Mom, Francine, was born in 1932. She had an older sister, Sheila, who was born in 1927. They were both born in Brooklyn. My grandparents were Yetta and Sam, whom I called Gram and Pops. My great grandparents, Gram's parents, emigrated from Poland and didn't speak English. They passed away when I was young. I have their wedding picture, which is cool. Pops' parents never emigrated and were in what we used to call the old country (Russia). Gram was a housewife; Pops was a painter getting his lungs full of asbestos.

Gram decided show business was the path her daughters should take. Can you spell stage mother? I think she invented the term. Starting with ballet, then encouraging them to sing, act, and audition for parts in whatever was casting. I have a Polaroid of my Mom in a Playboy bunny costume from before I was born. I'm sure that must have thrilled Gram. Mom outlined her face with a pen. I always wondered why she did that and was angry that she "ruined" the picture. Perhaps she was embarrassed …?

When Mom was 21, she met and married my father, Nat. Mom had me nine months later. I was an only child. I was born in March 1954 at the French Hospital in Manhattan. I don't think my mother breastfed me. It wasn't fashionable at the time. Does it matter? Why even bring it up? Nowadays, research shows that breastfed babies tend to have better health later in life. That doesn't apply to me as I'm extremely healthy in my old age. Plus breastfeeding creates a bond between mother and baby. Perhaps that is why I don't remember Mom being particularly physically affectionate. I think I was conceived on the first night of her marriage to my dad. She denies it. Well, she's denied a lot of things. Later, I would chalk that up to dementia.

I'm a Pisces: for some, that will shed light on me and my personality. For others, I'm guessing they will scratch their head. In a nutshell, Pisces is known for being creative in various arenas—painting, performing, writing, etc. They are also known for problems with their feet. Pisces are smart, creative, and deeply intuitive and can be close to psychic. They feel things deeply and have incredibly strong gut reactions. A Pisces "knows" things from deep within and is intelligent. A Pisces has a profound respect for the power of the human mind. Albert Einstein was a Pisces. Those characteristics describe me, especially the feet, not the Einstein part; I wish.

The thing about being intuitive is that you must be open to it, which I am. In my opinion, most people are head-blind. In the '90s, I catered for Char Margolis, a world-famous psychic, for her book launch, *Questions from Earth, Answers from Heaven*. She told Kelly Rippa she was pregnant on air before Kelly told her boss/producer. Oops.

I believe in the law of attraction. I believe in karma. I believe I am living proof of both. I know I have spirit guides. I feel them in my soul and my gut. Things happen, and I know it is how it should be. Or that I'm on the right track. Or I'll think of someone, and the phone rings or I get a text from them. And vice versa. I will call someone, and they say, "I was JUST thinking about you." Char teaches people how to tap into their intuition, and I'm a good student. I always had a gut feeling about things, even as a kid.

Mom was a June Taylor dancer on *The Jackie Gleason Show*, second from the left, which was how you were identified. They were like the Rockettes. Both were dancing drill teams. The only difference was The Rockettes performed on stage at Radio City Music Hall in New York City and the June Taylor Dancers performed on TV. I do remember sitting in front of the television and watching her dance when I was a tiny baby. It sounds unbelievable, and maybe I'm hallucinating, but I swear I remember. Most people nowadays haven't a clue who Jackie Gleason was or who the June Taylor Dancers were. The dancers were on *What's My Line*, a game show, in 1956, and the person who posted it on YouTube was kind enough to give me a copy and allowed me to post it on my YouTube. I don't have many other recollections until I was about four or five when we lived in West Nyack, upstate New York. Nat was a used car sales manager. He sold Fiats, Saabs, and Volvos before anyone knew what they were. Later, it was Volkswagens (VWs or Bugs). His claim to fame in our house was sitting on the pot reading trashy paperbacks.

We lived in a nice, two-story house. I remember the house for a few things. The first thing was throwing all my toys out the window for my friends and neighbors. Yep, I was the definition of precocious.

Another thing I remember is the stage-like area, where I would dance around to music on the record player. Paul Anka was my all-time favorite singer and my absolute idol. Little did I know then that he'd become more than just a voice on vinyl to me. When I met him years later, the cocktail of emotions that swept over me was overwhelming when he approached me to say hello. I was ecstatic, elated, horrified, excited, thrilled, overjoyed, jubilant, delirious, stoked, and speechless. The floodgate of tears burst.

Another thing I remember about that house was eating chewable vitamins until I puked. Hey, I was hungry. My parents weren't around. Needless to say, they were not amused when they found out.

The house also held sad memories of my parents' fights and screaming matches, mostly about money. And like many young children of divorce, I believed it was my fault. Perhaps Nat couldn't make enough as a used car salesman to support his young family, which put Mom under pressure to audition and find acting jobs.

When the divorce finally happened, I remember feeling ... relief. No more screaming, no more slammed doors. But even at seven, I knew what came next: choosing sides. I hated it. My dad wasn't around much, but I still wanted him in my life. My mom, on the other hand, wanted him gone—completely. And I was caught in the middle, too young to understand why love could turn into war.

Gram was the epitome of a "stage mother." It seemed every ounce of attention, affection, and praise went to Aunt Sheila. It made sense that Aunt Sheila won the seventh annual Tony for Best Actress in *Wish You Were Here*, and my Mom was "just" a chorus girl. This is not to say Mom didn't have her own impressive credits. She understudied Barbra (need I say a last name?) in her first show, *I Can Get It for You Wholesale*, in 1962. I remember Barbra playing with me as if I were her little doll. She would put a fall (called extensions now) on my head and make up my face. I wish I had a picture. She only had a son, Jason. Maybe she wished she had a daughter?

Actors are constantly auditioning. When my Mom did work, I remember being left with black maids. When I saw the film *The Help*, it resonated deeply with me. Nowadays, these caregivers are called nannies or housekeepers.

When I was three or four, and we didn't have—or couldn't afford—a housekeeper, my mom left me with our Asian neighbors, who had young children. They were home-schooling them, so I learned to read and write before most kids. I wasn't allowed to watch cartoons; I was allowed to read books. People are amazed when I tell them I never saw animated films like *Bambi* or *101 Dalmatians*.

I'm sure Mom did the best she could. In my opinion, I always felt she was super critical and judgmental, which she learned from her mother. If I parted my hair in the middle or on the side, she would rather I pull it back in a ponytail. My mom, bless her soul, never let me pick out my own clothes. It wasn't just about looking good—it was about being perfect. She would sigh in frustration if I so much as parted my hair the 'wrong' way. Every outfit had to be carefully curated, as if I were walking a red carpet instead of just going to school. Everything had to be perfectly coordinated, with colors that matched just right. At the time, I didn't question it or try to rebel. But now, I wonder—was it love? Or was it her way of controlling the one thing in her life that she could control: me? That stuck with me into adulthood—so when I see people in mismatched outfits or out in their pajamas, I can't help but cringe. She had a certain set of standards that she passed down to me, and for that, I'm forever grateful. But if I'm being honest, I wouldn't mind a little less rigidity in my own beliefs and way of thinking. It makes me wonder about the whole **Nature vs. Nurture** debate—the ongoing question of whether we're shaped more by genetics or by the environment we grow up in. Are my perfectionist tendencies something I was born with, or did my mother's meticulous standards program them into me? Maybe it's both. Maybe we inherit certain traits but reinforce them through experience. Either way, it's a hard habit to break. Now, I feel the pull of judgment every waking moment. And I fight it.

As I got older, my Mom wasn't happy with my nose. When I hit my tween and teen years, she was eager for me to get it "fixed." I remember thinking, "But I look like Barbra." Nevertheless, she found one of the top plastic surgeons in Manhattan, Dr. Howard Diamond. And I got it fixed.

I don't blame her for anything. What good would that do? I just never wanted to "be" like her. As I watch all the social media, I wonder, "How can people take selfies with a nose like that?" Then I think you are horrible! I'm trying to make a point. At least I'm mindful of it. And I must keep fighting it. And I do. And I will. I dislike being judgmental.

1956

As soon as I could walk, or maybe before, I was placed on the back of a pony. That was the beginning of my lifelong obsession with horses. Horses didn't judge. They didn't care if my hair was parted wrong or if I had the perfect nose. They just existed—strong, beautiful, free. I think that's why I was obsessed with them. In a world where I felt scrutinized at every turn, a horse only cared if you were kind and knew how to hold the reins.

A horse gets to know you by smelling your breath when you blow into its nose like dogs sniff your hand to get acquainted. Well, that was all I had to know. I exchanged breath with every beautiful equine nose I could find after that. There were a lot of horse-drawn carriages in Manhattan, so I was pretty busy. I liked to think the horses knew that I was one of them.

My favorite TV show was *Fury*, the story of a horse and a boy named Joey who loved him. Fury was a black stallion I yearned to meet or own. He knelt so Joey could mount him and ride without a bridle, which is not an easy feat. Years later ('79) I had a new love: the *Black Stallion* film. I bought the DVD. I swear I love animals more than people. Move over, Betty White. I know you are hanging out at the Rainbow Bridge with all the animals who are waiting for their people.

1957

When I was three years old, I managed to escape the confines of my crib and fell hard and broke my right elbow. At that age, bones are still mostly cartilage, and the doctor said he couldn't set it until I was older. When I was about six or seven years old, the doc decided it was time to fix it. He had to break it again and put my arm in a cast that I wore for what felt like an eternity but was in actuality six months.

The day they took the cast off—before I even had the chance to enjoy the freedom of two functioning arms—one of my relatives decided to chase me, and I fell and broke that same elbow again. My poor Gram was beside herself. She was so furious that she never spoke to that woman again. That one fall didn't just break my arm—it fractured the relationship between them forever. And for months, I had to go back to the doc so he could make sure it had set correctly and I had full motion.

The '60s

Mom and Nat ultimately separated and, thankfully, divorced when I was seven, finally. People often stay together for their child's sake, but in my opinion, that's unfortunate.

Mom started dating, and one of the gentlemen wanted to take her to a film screening. She couldn't find a sitter for me, but her date didn't mind my coming along with them.

At the screening, we bumped into a production assistant for Meredith Willson, who was casting and getting ready to direct a Broadway show called *Here's Love*. It was an adaptation of the film *Miracle on 34th Street*. He was casting Natalie Wood's part, Susan Walker. People said I resembled Natalie. I wish.

He looked at me and asked my mother if I could sing and dance. "Of course!" was the reply. When you are an actor, it always must be "Yes, I can do that!" And no, I didn't sing, and no, I didn't dance. Thus, I commenced intensive lessons before the audition. And they were muy painful.

I was not talented in my opinion and had to practice constantly to keep my vocal and physical muscles in shape. Mom decided "Hey Look Me Over" and "Red, Red Robin" would be my songs.

I got the part. My mom insisted my stage name be Bond—just like hers and Aunt Sheila's. I was mentioned in every major newspaper and *Time Magazine*. Clippings are in the book *When We Wrote Letters, The Sixties, Volume 1* (available on Amazon).

Mom asked her dear friend, Jackie Susann, to be my godmother and mentor. It was a "thing." A godmother (or father) helped you navigate "show biz" and the process, which was an important aspect of building a successful career. Jackie was the author of *Valley of the Dolls*, her debut novel, published in 1966. It was a runaway bestseller upon release and remains one of the best-selling novels ever.

Then I got fired. The conversation went something like this: They asked me to rehearse. I said, "Why? I know my lines." They said, "Don't let the door hit your behind on the way out." Just like that. Hmmm. Do I hold the record for being the youngest person ever fired? I searched the internet and couldn't find anything to substantiate this claim.

I remember walking out of that theater, dazed, like I'd been slapped. My mom didn't say a word as we left, just marched ahead, her heels clicking furiously against the pavement. When we got home, I half-expected a lecture, but she just sat down, lit a cigarette, and stared off into the distance. That was worse. I wanted her to yell, to be angry—at them, at me, at something. But the silence hung between us, thick with disappointment.

Gram and Pops were proud of my accomplishments and loved to show me off. They used to parade me around their apartment complex in Rego Park and made me sing and dance for their neighbors.

Next, I got hired to do an M&M commercial. "Melts in your mouth, not in your hands." There were two little girls; I was the tall one. It was supposedly the longest-running national M&M commercial. After numerous takes, they gave us a bucket to spit out the candy so we wouldn't get sick eating so much of it. Afterward, when it was on the air, whoever was watching TV at the time, either Mom or me, would start screaming, "It's on!" and the other would come running into the room to watch. Then, I got a week-long part on a soap, *The Doctors*. Next, I sang on an album with the Singing Nun, and I had to sing in French.

1962-63

I think Nat loved dogs as much as I did. I can't say more than I did, as NO ONE loved dogs more than me. We had a GSD (German shepherd dog) bitch Cindy. She was well-trained, but in those days, it entailed roughness, unlike today. The results were evident with endless commands of "Sit!" and "Sit, stay!" Nat could go into McDonald's and place her in a sit-stay while he went inside for food, and she wouldn't move a muscle. The customers entering and leaving were wary, but she didn't move. He bred her and sold her pups. The first two litters, she had nine puppies, and in the last litter, she had seven.

Each time, after the pups were weaned, I would latch onto the runt female, kinda like the puppies latched onto the teat. I looked at my dad with soulful, hazel eyes and asked, "Can we keep this one? And name her Betsy? Pretty please with sugar on top?" The first two times, the answer was "No," then, the third time, he said, "YES!" My heart leaped for joy. After Mom and Nat separated, he moved into his own apartment— taking the dogs with him. That broke my heart.

I stood in the doorway, watching them disappear, my face hot with anger. They were my dogs, too. Didn't I get a say? That was the moment I realized that in divorce, kids aren't the only ones who lose things. Sometimes, you lose the ones you love the most—even if they have four legs.

After Cindy and Betsy, he got another female he named Mindy. Three German shepherds in an apartment in Manhattan? Yep. Then he moved to DC into a first-floor apartment with a small yard and chain link fence. He got a boy, Smokey, to have a stud handy. People would pass by and torment and tease them so they would bite the fence. A few teeth were lost.

I attended a public school in Manhattan for third grade, PS 87. I don't remember a thing about it. I just remember what a dork I looked like.

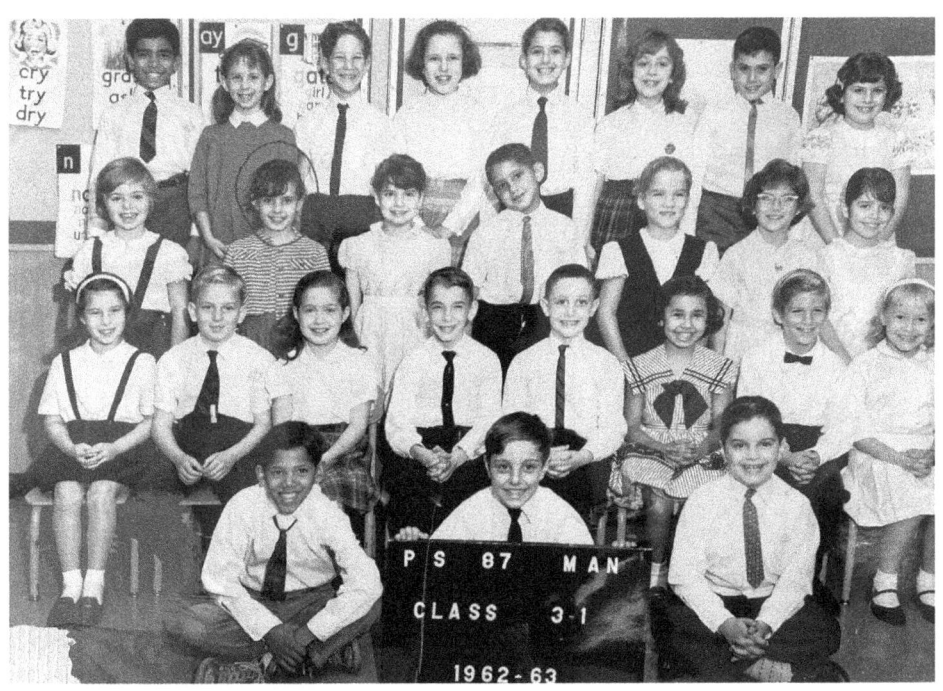

1965

In fourth and fifth grade, while I was acting, I went to PCS, Professional Children's School. It was a school for kids who had to audition, rehearse, work, etc. Wikipedia says: "Professional Children's School is a not-for-profit, college preparatory school geared toward working and aspiring child actors and dancers in grades six through twelve. The school was founded in New York City in 1914 to provide an academic education to young people working on the stage, in

Vaudeville, or 'on the road.'" I recently discovered that Aunt Sheila also went to PCS!

At PCS, I met and flirted with Demetri, 12, a sweet, talented Greek pianist prodigy. He was madly in love with me. Well, we were tweens, so how madly could it be? So was Fred, also 12, an accomplished guitar prodigy who trained under Segovia, the preeminent guitarist of that era. I was a little hussy and a major flirt.

I got mostly As and Bs in the subjects I liked (reading and writing), Cs in the ones I didn't like or wasn't good at (science, math), and a D in citizenship. I was always a troublemaker. I rode the bus alone to get to school and was in love with a bus driver who was a Buddy Hackett doppelgänger. That was "my type" —old men who looked like my Pops, my grandfather, the sweetest human on the planet. I think I was always searching for love. Buddy was in a Broadway show with Aunt Sheila in 1954, a comedy called *Lunatics and Lovers.*

I feel bad for kids today who can't even step outside without a chaperone hovering nearby.

I'm not sure if there is more crime against kids now or if social media is making us more aware of it. It's a different time now. I'm also sad for the children who can't be without their devices or spend one minute engaged in conversation, walking, eating, or doing anything. How will these kids get along in the world or have a conversation?

Mom and I moved to a little one-bedroom apartment on West 75th Street over Stark's Restaurant. Nat didn't pay alimony or child support, which didn't sit well with Mom. How can you blame her? She needed to keep a roof over our heads and feed us. I remember MANY cockroaches—screaming and squealing and trying to bat them with a rolled-up newspaper. I don't believe they could be avoided in an apartment in Manhattan.

There was a candy store on the ground floor and Nat got me a charge account there, so I was never without whatever they sold (candy? ice cream? And my FAVORITE: cream sodas?)

Perhaps he thought that would make up for not giving Mom money.

He always brought me *Archie* comic books that I read and collected diligently. Ultimately, I gave the comics to the kids in the Children's Hospital. If I had those now, I'd be a millionaire, literally.

Nat would also bring me a Barbie or Ken doll or accessory almost every time he saw me. Boy, that was an area of contention. Mom hated that he brought me presents. Perhaps she thought he was trying to compensate for not giving child support. She kept nothing to herself. She was always bitching about him, which made me extremely uncomfortable. It was like she needed me to hate him too, to erase any memories I had of him. But I couldn't. She wanted me to see only the bad, but love doesn't work like that.

I never saw the Barbies after we moved, and I was getting older, so I didn't think about them or miss them. In later years, when I asked Mom where they were, she said she had them "somewhere." If I had them today, they would have also made me a millionaire since I took really good care of them.

One day, when Nat came to visit, Mom wouldn't let me out of the apartment to see him. No child support, no visitation was her new motto. There was a lot of pushing and shoving, but I won. I got her out of the way, opened the door, and ran into his arms.

I was never made, or shall I say encouraged, to drink milk. So, at a very young age, I ended up needing nine cavities filled at once, under gas (nitrous oxide). Gram's brother, Uncle Harry, was my dentist. My love of nitrous is powerful to this day.

Mom started dating George Smith. He was Jewish. People would ask, "Jewish? With a name like Smith?" Turns out, when his ancestors arrived at Ellis Island, their surname was Kowal—which means "blacksmith" in Polish. Immigration officials simply said, "Smith, next."

Mom and George married when I was nine, and we moved from West 75th Street to East 72nd Street. Just like the song: movin' on up, to the East Side, to a deluxe apartment in the sky. Well, it was only the eleventh floor. We finally got a piece of the pie. Believe me when I say a WORLD of difference in Manhattan. With his astute business acumen, George oversaw my career, a role he excelled in. He was a serial entrepreneur.

His friends owned a restaurant upstate called Spindletop. They had racehorses; it was a branding thing. George bought a trotter as an investment and told me he bought ME a trotter. That's just the way he was—kind, thoughtful, and loving.

When you live in Manhattan and are well-to-do, your parents ship you off to summer camp every year. The first one I went to was Camp Tamarack, a Western riding camp. My best bud was Jamie. We both had red cowboy boots. We raced barrels and got in trouble as much as 11-year-olds could. Recently, she tracked me down, and we reestablished our friendship. I am the one who usually tries to find people from my past. At first, I didn't remember her, but when she mentioned the red cowboy boots, it all came flooding back.

After Tamarack, I went to Camp Wishe in Middletown, NY, about an hour and a half out of the city. I switched to English riding because, in Manhattan, you rarely saw cowboys riding with Western saddles in Central Park.

In February, I started getting ready for camp! I sewed my name tags into my clothes. Never mind that camp wasn't until summer. By the time May rolled around, I was at the curb tapping my foot, waiting to get my trunk into the car and leave.

George owned Duval, an ice cream factory, and about mid-summer, he sent an ice cream truck to camp for everyone; I was the SHEro of all time—who doesn't love ice cream?

George wanted to adopt me and make me his heiress, his beneficiary, and Nat said, "Sure." They both always wanted what was best for me. So, George did. And we all lived happily ever after. The end. KIDDING. Nat remarried and had two kids.

Gram got Parkinson's. Mom was impatient because Gram couldn't walk normally and instead shuffled slowly due to the disease. I cringed when I heard Mom speak to her mother. Gram also developed breast cancer. I don't remember what year she died. Ditto Pops. Pops was a painter. I think he died of a lung ailment due to inhaling asbestos.

George suffered a heart attack, a wake-up call that life couldn't continue at its frantic New York pace. He and Mom, wanting a change and a chance to heal, decided to move to Mexico for a year. They hoped the slower rhythm of life there would give him a chance to escape the relentless rat race that consumed him living in the city. It was a bold move, driven by the need to reclaim health and rediscover peace. He sold Duval to Dolly Madison so we could move.

1966

George, Mom, and I moved to Cuernavaca, Mexico, when I was 12 years old and in seventh grade. My parents enrolled me in Joan Werner's American School. George got me a horse! We found a pinto horse, named Hormiga, which means ant in Spanish. At first, she had no idea what carrots or apples were. She might not have ever been ridden because when I tried to put on her saddle, the bucking would start. After a bunch of good meals and a whole lot of love, we became best buds. She allowed me to saddle and ride her. I was careful not to betray her trust, yank on her mouth or dig my heels into her.

I was a good student. I mainly got 90s, two 80s, and three 100s, and I still have my report card to prove it. That's how I felt I got love from my parents—good grades! I learned Spanish in three months. I still speak Spanglish to this day—kinda sorta. Spanglish, yes, it's a movie and a language.

George and Mom rented a huge villa with live-in caretakers when we arrived. You needed roller skates to get from one end of the estate to the other. I think the caretakers were not happy they had to start working for the "gringos." They had been living there alone for a while.

One day, I fell off a wall at school and broke my right pointer finger. A male teacher took my hand into his two big ones to make a human splint until I could get real medical help. There are not a ton of things I remember in detail, but this was one moving memory I'll never forget.

1967

We moved back to Manhattan after the school year ended. George got me a Kerry Blue Terrier. I named him Sean. They sent me to Miss Hewitt's, a prestigious, private girl's school in New York City's Upper East Side. It was renowned for its rigorous academics and commitment to nurturing future leaders. The school fosters a high-achievement culture, empowering girls to excel academically and develop strong leadership skills. We wore uniforms—I'll never forget the dark green and black plaid skirts and knee socks. We had to have our skirts below our knees. So, of course, we hiked them up from the waist until a good amount of thigh was visible. I don't understand why as there was never a boy in sight.

In eighth grade, we studied Latin. I remember some of the girls a grade ahead of me did drugs. I was the biggest goody two shoes, standing on a pedestal preaching about the evils of drugs. Maybe I was a precursor to Nancy Reagan.

1968

Camp Wishe

Sleepaway riding camp, and all that entailed, was the best time of my young life, maybe my whole life. It was heaven. I loved it all—bungalows, campfires, swimming, riding, jumping, dressage, drill team, tennis, fencing, crafts, singalongs, first aid, scuba, lifesaving course, mucking stalls, brushing and washing the horses, and swimming with them. You name it, we did it! I was a camper the first year and the next year became a

CIT (counselor in training.) After that, you can become a counselor, but that wasn't in the cards for me.

My favorite horses were Mascara, Rockney, and Cherry. My closest friends were Anita and Cora. I stumbled upon a Facebook (FB) page for Wishers (ladies who went to Camp Wishe). I found bunkmates and counselors I went to camp with. No sooner had I found Cora than she passed away. That sucked.

I had a girl crush on a stunning woman named Yogi. She was gorgeous. The Wishes were an incredible family, and their daughter DeeDee was a phenomenal rider who seemed born in the saddle. Grandma Wishe cooked with a team of helpers, creating meals that brought everyone together. DeeDee's horse, Pawnee, was the best in the entire stable. We all idolized DeeDee, mesmerized by her talent, and dreamed of riding Pawnee. But Pawnee was no ordinary horse, and only the most skilled riders were ever granted the honor of riding her. For the rest of us, simply watching them together was enough to inspire awe.

Camp lasted for eight weeks. At the end of each summer, there was a horse show where parents came to pick up the kids so we could show them what we learned for their money. It was typically the Saturday before Labor Day. I won first place out of all the campers.

Then we did drill team to REALLY impress them. The last year I went, Anita fell off her horse and got a concussion, even though she was wearing a riding helmet. She was hospitalized and in a coma for four days. She seemed to recover fully, but later developed epilepsy. She wanted to share her story with the world so that people would not be afraid of epilepsy, and she ended up passing away far too soon.[1]

---

1 https://purpledayeveryday.org/anita-kaufmann-foundation/

1969

A cousin, thinking it would be funny, taught me to smoke when I was just ten years old. By the time I was 15, I had been smoking long enough that the fear of dying from lung cancer consumed me. Depression and anxiety took over most of my preteen and teenage years. George made sure I spent time soaking in a hot bath, hoping that it would ease my anxiety. It rarely did.

Writing letters was huge back then. I remember my parents opening and reading my mail. They never admitted it, but I think they did it so they could find out what I was up to and what kind of trouble I was in or was going to be in. That's probably when I developed major trust issues. I think I've grown out of them. I hope so.

We had a big old Cadillac convertible, which I called "the boat." For vacations, usually during spring break, we'd drive down to Florida, singing show tunes all the way. George's favorite song was "Fly Me to the Moon," and he had an amazing voice!

I went to Miss Hewitt's with a Thai girl, Yinglak, Yui for short, and P-Yui to relatives. Yui's parents owned the largest Thai-speaking newspaper in Bangkok. Yui's family sent their children to boarding schools in America for education. They sent one to Dallas, one to LA, one to Denver, and sent Yui to NYC. Then, they could bring back all they had learned in America to run their empire.

Mom and George had a passion for traveling so, during their absences, I would board at Hewitt's. Over time, Yui and I developed a deep and meaningful friendship. As eighth grade came to an end, her parents extended an invitation to her classmates for a summer trip to Thailand. All we had to do was buy a plane ticket; they would handle the rest. Besides myself, only one other girl, Katie (whom I also recently reconnected with on Facebook), was up for the adventure.

The moment we landed, we were quickly swept up in a whirlwind of activities, following Pa's jam-packed schedule as the owner of the largest Thai-speaking newspaper. Every day was filled with events, and we quickly adapted to the fast-paced rhythm of his work. At one event, I watched him take a small Thai chili and eat it—no food, just the chili. As soon as he finished, he wiped his brow, clearly feeling the full force of the chili's heat. I had never cared for spicy food, so I was beyond amazed watching him do it.

While my parents had hoped the experience would ease my anxiety, it ended up having the exact opposite effect. The plan was to stay the entire summer. I ended up flying home alone after just three weeks. I remember sitting in that airport staring at the departure board like it held all the answers. I felt like I was unraveling. Every day had been too fast, too loud, too much. I couldn't keep up, and I didn't want to. All I wanted was to go home, to my bed, to something that felt safe.

When I got home? More hot baths. Yui and I remained good friends for a long time, and I visited her in Bangkok two more times. And thankfully grew out of the panic attacks so I could enjoy Thailand! I've literally been around the world three times, which is pretty cool when I think about it and seeing so many different cultures. The last time I visited Yui, spicy food had become a favorite and I requested it at nearly every meal. She looked at me with incredulity and said, "What did you do with my friend Sheri?"

The '70s

It was important to Mom and George that I was smarter than other kids. They thought it would be wonderful for me to join Mensa, the world's largest and oldest high-IQ society. It is a non-profit organization open to people who score at the 98th percentile or higher on a standardized, supervised IQ test. I scored 138, the 94th percentile, so I didn't make it. I always felt like a disappointment to them. I didn't feel "almost good enough." I felt like a failure. Every time

Mensa came up, I imagined them shaking their heads thinking: "if only she'd scored higher". They never said it, but sometimes, silence says everything.

Even with his lifestyle changes, George's bad heart still plagued him. But slowing down? Not a chance. He was a serial entrepreneur—always hustling, always working. Although I'm not his biological child, I definitely inherited his entrepreneurial gene. Mom and he decided it was time to experience a more laid-back atmosphere so they decided we should move to Las Vegas.

I had just completed tenth grade at Hewitt's and had I graduated from there, I would have been able to attend the college of my choice due to the high standards of the school. But that was not to be. When we got to Vegas, I went to Valley High for eleventh and twelfth grades. In Vegas, there was very little for kids to do, albeit drugs. It was a different culture in Vegas. Most kids drove. In Manhattan, there was no need.

My new friends wasted no time introducing Miss Goody Two Shoes to drugs. First up?

Psilocybin—the trippy little fungi that makes you see God, or at least neon lights in a whole new way. They took me down Fremont Street in a convertible. I sat in the back seat, tripping on the lights. It felt like the whole city was alive—pulsing, breathing, winking just for me. The neon signs weren't just lights; they were messages. Messages I'd never quite decode, but in that moment, I was sure they meant something. Is it a wonder I gave up caring about school or college? I think I fried my brain by experimenting with and doing drugs.

When we got to Vegas, George got me another horse. Hormiga was in Mexico, mostly forgotten. I don't remember the horse's name, but I remember the friend I used to ride with. One day, she was tripping on LSD (acid) and rode around naked. I found her on FB but didn't mention this incident. What happens in Vegas …?

One night I had a date with a hippie who sported a huge blond afro. He came over to pick me up, and George took our picture. We weren't even out the door when he whispered, "First and last, you won't see him again." I lost my virginity to him that night. A rebellious: "I'll show you, Dad!" moment. Looking back? Maybe not my finest hour. Yes, at the time I thought I was a horrible person and a horrible daughter. I never saw the guy again.

As soon as I turned sixteen, I moved out and started living with a bunch of hippies in a commune, for lack of a better term. I remember drinking beer for lunch. Beer has wheat, right? That's a food group, isn't it? I thought beer had nutritional value, and since I couldn't afford much to eat, at least I got a buzz for my money. I don't remember if there was sex, but I assume there must have been.

As usual, George tried to help me. He got me a job with his friend who owned a drycleaning store. That lasted for a minute—and I never exaggerate. I don't know if anyone could have saved me at that point. I was lost. I drifted between parties, bad decisions, and whatever felt good in the moment. A job? A future? Those weren't on my radar.

Another job I had was that of a box girl (box person?) at a supermarket. Eventually, I had to move back home. I couldn't make enough money to support myself.

George was always a string-puller. The best string he ever pulled for me was a lifeguard job at Caesars Palace. It was like a Manhattan apartment—you had to die to get one. I was in love with my boss, and a co-worker was in love with me. Isn't that always the way?

My Mom had a million-year-old mink jacket. Again, I NEVER exaggerate. I talked her into giving it to me, and I had it made into a mink bikini. I wore it at work, and all the guys (guests and co-workers) at Caesars' pool went wild. Their partners, dates, or spouses then went wild on them. I'm glad I could help, ladies.

1972

I graduated high school on June 8th and panicked. How I got a diploma is a mystery since I don't remember doing a bloody thing my senior year. I'd gotten good grades my whole life without even trying, or so it seemed. I thought, *Now what? What do I do with my life?*

I was back in my parents' house, and soon it became the same as it ever was—difficult and tricky—constant conflicts and fighting. We just couldn't seem to get along. My mother often criticized my choices, making me question my abilities and worth. After working several jobs that would last for what seemed like five minutes, I knew I needed to be an entrepreneur like George, whatever that meant.

I had no idea how to start. Then I had a brilliant idea. I'd join the military. My parents were nonplussed. Dad said, "Sure, as long as you join the elite branch," and I thought, "Hmmm, I never even knew there was an elite branch." His idea was the Air Force since he had served in that branch. I said Navy, which was acceptable to him. "You're in the Navy now. You're not behind a plow, you'll never get rich, you son of a bitch, you're in the Navy now."

1973

January 12

I left for boot camp in Orlando, Florida and got through eight grueling weeks. The males and females were segregated by chain-link fences. I flirted with every male in sight. I remember one guy was Bryce. We had immediate and intense attraction. We exchanged addresses and corresponded relentlessly. We finally found a way to connect in the real world. I think we were planning to get married. Say what? Me? Ha-ha!

Fun fact: in those days, you had to put your social security number ON THE ENVELOPE for mail to get to you. Crazy, huh? I went home on leave for two weeks. Mom and George were playing golf and owning or starting a business as usual. I managed to meet and fall in love with my first true love, Teddy. His folks were from Ohio and owned a junkyard; I lovingly referred to him as my junkyard dog. He was gorgeous, and a mechanic who worked hard. He always had greasy hands stained from working on car engines that I wanted all over me all the time. We had major lust. I didn't sleep the first three days we were together; we had constant sex, and that was all I could think about. Then, it was time to leave for Hospital Corp School in Great Lakes, and I could barely tear myself away. But I did; I had no choice.

What was the Navy like? Don't ask. Ok, I'll tell ya. Picture the film *Private Benjamin* on steroids. "I have to march at what time?" Insert 5 a.m., if I'm not mistaken. Which meant getting up BEFORE that to dress, brush teeth, make bed, etc. We had to clean the bathroom, especially the toilets, spotless with a toothbrush. Uniforms had to be impeccable. Shirts had to be ironed, shoes spit-shined, and hair neatly pulled back if it was long.

It became apparent that my bunkmates' strengths varied. Consequently, we adopted a strategy where each person focused on their particular strength, ensuring efficient and effective teamwork. One person would spit shine (all the shoes), one iron (all the clothes), one make all the beds, one cleaned all the toilets, etc.

After I got out of the Navy, I went back to Vegas and moved in with Teddy. But that wasn't meant to last. My Mom and George didn't have a clue how to deal with me when I returned, so they got in touch with Nat. Nat had been battling lung cancer for seven years. They decided I should move to Long Beach, Long Island, to be with him since he didn't have much time left. I agreed, and he agreed. He had a new wife, a five-year-old daughter, a three-year-old son, and Betsy, my dog before I left to explore the world. At this time, she was about 13 years old and nearing the end of her life.

Coming from Vegas, I had no warm coat for freezing and snowy New York. The first thing Nat did was buy me a suede and sheepskin coat that I can still picture in my mind's eye. He also bought me a car—Herbie the Love Bug. That was so sweet. As his pain worsened, we spent many evenings at bars, trying to numb it by drinking too much. Given my addictive personality, keeping up with him was easy. Back then, there was a lot of uncertainty about how cancer developed, spread, or whether it was contagious. He was extremely cautious, refusing to let anyone drink from his glass or use his eating utensils. I didn't have the scientific facts, but I never believed it worked that way.

December 8

I worked as a server at a bar in Connecticut called Gulliver's. I don't remember how I got the job or why I was traveling so far from home in Long Beach. I drove there every weekend in my bug. On that night, I had a car accident on the way to work. Some person coming in the opposite direction crossed the center divider and wiped me out. The driver's side of my little VW was demolished. I had a contusion from my left hip to my knee. After the accident, I never went back to Gulliver's.

1974

January 3

I was in Long Beach Hospital for surgery to address some female health issues when I met Garry, a high-strung, Type A stockbroker dealing with his own challenges. From the moment we crossed paths, we were drawn to each other like magnets, an undeniable connection sparking between us. I wrote to George, "I met a wonderful guy," and he wrote back saying Garry sounded great. And in the beginning, I guess he was. We moved in together, and since Garry made a good living, I naively hoped he would "take care of me," making life feel a little less like a struggle. But his true nature soon emerged. Before long, he became controlling, threatening, and violent. I never told my parents when things changed.

June 30

I found out Gullivers burned down and a bunch of my friends were killed in the fire. I always wonder, had I not had the car accident, would I have still worked there? I could have been inside that night. It's eerie to think about the way life pushes you off one path and onto another. Survivor's guilt? I concluded God must have something for me to do or finish down here.

1975

March 20

The last week of Nat's life was agonizing. Watching him deteriorate from cancer, enduring unbearable pain, tore my heart out. That week led up to my birthday, March 19. Mom, George, and Nat's wife all told me, "Don't go to the hospital today; it's your birthday." Nat might've been in a coma at that point, so they felt he wouldn't know one way or the other. Really? But what if he did? What if he was waiting for me? Holding on just a little longer waiting to see me again to say his final goodbye?

I've always regretted not going to see him that day. He left this world at 2 a.m., the morning after my birthday. I can't help but feel he held on so he wouldn't pass on my birthday. Draw your own conclusion.

His wife gave me his pajamas, and the hospital gave me the sheepskins they'd used under him to prevent bedsores. Holding them, I felt both comforted and devastated; these were the last pieces of him I'd ever have. I knew I would keep and cherish them forever, reminders of the moments we shared in those final days.

Even after Nat died, I couldn't quit cigarettes. I loved my cigarettes and continued smoking for the next 30 or so years. It took me three times, using the drug Chantix, before I was able to quit. You're only supposed to take it once. And that wasn't the only tool I needed to use to quit. There was also a plethora of gum, straws, hard candy, toothpicks, hypnosis tapes, and every other trick or suggestion I could find or try.

After Nat passed, I moved out of his house and got my own place in Great Neck, a town near Long Beach, so I could stay close to his family and Betsy and drive into the city to audition. I thought I was supposed to be an actor and took acting lessons with Lee Strasberg. He said I was talented, and I hoped he was right. One day, Nat's wife called me, frantic, saying that Betsy couldn't get up. "What should I do?" There was nothing she could do. It was Betsy's time. She joined Dad soon thereafter. I know she died of a broken heart, regardless of her old age.

April 26

Garry and I got married. Not long after, I got pregnant and decided to have an abortion. I felt no guilt, no remorse. I knew with every fiber of my being that I wasn't meant to be a mother. Not with Garry. Not with anyone. The world was already messy enough—why bring a child into it? So, I made it permanent. I got fixed like every cat or dog should. And I've never looked back.

1976

Garry and I moved to Centre Island on Long Island's North Shore. Centre Island is located within the town of Oyster Bay in Nassau County, New York. At the time, this village was known for several notable residents, including musician Billy Joel, lyricist Alan Jay Lerner, media tycoon Rupert Murdoch, and political commentator Sean Hannity. And then there was us.

In those days, the sand and beaches around us, from Oyster Bay to Long Island Sound, were rich with vast amounts of clams and oysters. A Pisces like me could not help but be in heaven. Garry went to the shore and came back with buckets overflowing with shellfish. He had an impressive talent for using his toes to extract them from the sand.

He'd put the buckets all around the kitchen floor, and I'd spend hours, if not days, dealing with them—cleaning, shucking, cooking, freezing, and giving them to friends and relatives.

Our property was amazing and spacious and my inner gardener emerged. I went crazy planting and growing vegetables. Garry used to say it cost me $30 for a cucumber or any of the vegetables with all the seeds, starts, fertilizer, and time I spent growing them.

At the time, brokerage firms gave stockbrokers a bonus to join their team and bring their clients. Garry switched jobs quicker than you could blink. We bought a boat and named her "Thank you, Paine Webber." We did a lot of fishing on our little 17-foot motorboat. He took a picture of me lying on the grass with a crapload of fish all around me. Fluke and flounder. Pisces in her element. We bought a goat and brought it home in the back seat of the car. It was a Toggenburg, and we creatively named her Toggen. Hazel, Garry's mom, was an antique dealer. She was a dear, sweet lady. She gave me two German bisque baby dolls, which I cherished. I always wondered how this hothead with a quick temper came out of her.

On July 1, 1976, he bought me a brand new, white Datsun 280Z for $8,000. One day, he stood in front of it with a cinder block and threatened to smash the hood. I said, "You paid for it; go for it if you feel you must." He didn't; he just threatened to do it. He was a man of many threats. When he gave me a black eye, a friend had a moving truck at the house the next day, the minute he went to work in Manhattan. I took the dolls and the car with me.

September 23

After passing the NY State Emergency Medical Technician exam, I was eager to begin my career.

However, despite my qualifications, securing a position as an EMT proved challenging. In the 1970s, emergency medical services were predominantly male-dominated, and women often faced significant barriers to entry. I continued to audition for acting roles. When those opportunities were scarce, I found work behind the camera in various productions. This behind-the-scenes work was a welcome change, as it lacked the stringent judgments on appearance that actors often faced. And a girl's gotta eat and pay bills.

I drove from Long Island into the city in my Z car, and I had a CB (citizens band radio). My handle was Mobile Medic. Back in this era, they were very popular with truckers to alert each other if there were smokies (cops) on the road to avoid tickets. I used to fly down the shoulder of the LIE (Long Island Expressway), so fast sometimes it's a wonder I never crashed or got caught. Like I said, I was a rebel. Ten-four, good buddy.

1977

Garry and I got divorced on November 9. I always said I was only married "for a minute," which was actually two whole years—it seemed like an eternity. I got custody of all our friends in the divorce, which was all that mattered. Shoutout to those people. Aloha Fran, Larry, and Laura. They are all still my friends to this day.

I auditioned for a small part with a few lines in the *Greek Tycoon*. I wasn't willing to sleep with one of the decision makers, but the girl who did sleep with him got the part with the lines. I *did* sleep with one of the other producers, and didn't find out until later that he was married. Then it was too late. I didn't notice the tan line on his wedding ring finger. Say what? Really, Captain Obvious? We were madly in lust. He lived in LA, and I was in NY, and we carried on a long-distance affair. After a while he decided he couldn't continue the affair long distance, so he told me to pack my bags and my cats and come to LA. I put a hitch on the back of my 280Z and rented a little trailer for my stuff. The cats were in the hatchback with their litter box and food. Fran sent her hubby, Larry, to drive with me to keep me safe. I was grateful for the company and co-driver. We made it to LA, and married producer had a house with a roommate situation set up for me in North Hollywood. He flew Larry back home.

1979

I appeared on *The Dating Game* and earned $22.50 for picking a bachelor from three contestants. I wore an outfit from Trashy Lingerie, a well-known lingerie store on La Cienega owned by Mitch and Tracy, which is still open in Hollywood. A few years ago, I stopped by to say hello, and they remembered me—I was probably their best customer back in the day.

I appeared on *The $100,000 Pyramid.* Unfortunately, I didn't win and didn't get paid anything, but I did receive flooring as a consolation prize. Since I didn't own a house or have anywhere to use it, I gaveit away.

The '80s

Married producer took me to the Cannes Film Festival—pretty heady stuff.

We saw lots of films, mingled with cool celebrities, and I took lots of pictures (with a CAMERA) like my life depended on it. One of my favorites? A shot of me taking a picture of … paparazzi taking a picture of me. This was not surprising since I wore a very provocative camisole, a matching micro-mini skirt, and fishnet stockings. Yes, Trashy again. And classic Cannes.

The affair with married producer was a textbook case and painfully predictable. He had a wife and child and claimed he was miserable and never slept with her. Yet he was by her side for important occasions (his birthday, for example) while I spent those same occasions alone, weeping. Eventually, they had another child (which had to be by immaculate conception, right?) Either way, science failed or he was the next coming of Joseph. I knew I had to end it. I just didn't know how to, gracefully or otherwise. Part of me clung to hope, wanting to believe he'd leave her, that I mattered enough. The logical part of me knew I was just the intermission between acts in his real life. I hated how small that made me feel.

Tax season time came. Like all good cheating husbands, he helped me with all aspects of my life. He took my documents so his accountant could do my taxes. His wife found them in his car. I wrote a letter to her and spilled my guts. I put it in the mail. I told him I had written it, and he said, "If the letter reaches her, we're done." I said, "Oh, thank God." I was thrust from having a protected life, trying to act, which didn't pay much or consistently, to being a person who had to get a "real" job … again.

After we broke up, I had a #MeToo which lasted about four weeks. For those living under a rock, #MeToo gained attention and recognition on social media in 2017 following the exposure of sexual abuse allegations against Harvey Weinstein. Mine looked like Tom Cruise and drove a navy Camaro. I blocked out his name, but I took a picture of him dressed in a suit in front of his car with Molly, my long-haired GSD. Details of his abuse are also blocked. I knew I was attracting this BS, and it had to stop! His name is gone, erased from my memory like a survival instinct. But there's the photo to remind me. A normal moment, frozen in time, but behind it? A month of darkness I don't fully let myself recall.

I know I didn't value myself (enough?) and was attracting these people and relationships. Although mine weren't sexual assault or rape, back in the day, let's just say I was propositioned a hell of a lot and probably touched when I didn't ask to be touched, in a way I didn't want to be touched. I just chalked it up to the way show business and Hollywood operated. That's what we were taught—this was the price of admission. Smile, laugh it off, don't make waves. But it chipped away at something inside me, something I wouldn't fully recognize until much later.

I started working at William Morris Agency (WMA) back when it truly operated as an agency. It has since evolved into something else and I'm not quite sure what. All the assistants sat outside their agents' offices as gatekeepers to the stars and the star makers. Abraham, a sweet Jewish boy, and I sat next to one another. It seemed like everyone was Jewish, did coke, and/ or was gay. Except perhaps for my boss Art, who was married, a straight arrow, and an anomaly in this landscape. Abraham died of HIV/AIDS. A lot of my co-workers, young gay men, died when this disease exploded on the scene at this time. I reconnected with Art on FB recently and then his wife messaged me on FB that he died.

My next #MeToo happened while I worked at WMA. One day, one of the *Star Trek* stars, my idol since 1965, came shuffling in. Since the show had ended, he couldn't get arrested (in the industry, that meant he couldn't get a job). So he came to see my boss, who was a TV packaging agent. He specialized in assembling creative elements—such as writers, producers, actors, and directors—for television shows or projects. They "package" these talents together and sell the complete project to networks or production companies. Somehow, he ended up at my apartment. He was married and tried to kiss me. Strangely, despite my past, this felt different. Maybe because he was my idol. My roomie at the time was my witness. Sadly she passed away, taking both my secret and my proof with her. I was so disillusioned by his advances that I transferred my idolization to one of the other stars. I will not name names. Why? It's not important to anyone except me.

As far back as I can remember, the dream of soaring through the sky like a bird had captivated my imagination. Flying wasn't just a dream—it was a feeling. A deep-seated belief that I was meant to lift off the ground, to escape, to be weightless.

The sensation of wind rushing past me, and seeing the sprawling scenery below were images burned into my mind for days after I had a flying dream. Someone once told me dreaming of flying often symbolizes freedom, ambition, or a desire to rise above challenges in waking life. How you feel during the flight—whether it's exhilarating or frightening—can also provide insight into how you feel about your current circumstances.

I heard that one of the first reality shows ever was casting. It was called *The Dream Thing*. The premise was simple yet captivating: make people's lifelong dreams come true while cameras rolled to capture the moment. Without hesitation, I submitted my application, pouring my heart out about my fervent desire to fly. I wanted to hang glide, suspended beneath a wing, relying on nothing but the wind to carry me. To my delight, I was selected.

As the day of filming approached, Mother Nature had other plans. The gusty winds and unpredictable air currents made hang gliding too dangerous. The producer, ever resourceful, quickly pivoted to Plan B: I was to fly a small prop plane. While I appreciated his efforts to salvage the situation, I couldn't help feeling a twinge of disappointment. Tim, the producer, was a very kind man. He made sure the hang gliding company gave me a chance to do it another day when the weather cooperated. I started working for him as PA (production assistant) and he became a dear friend for forty years. He loved me when I was totally unlovable. I found him years later on Facebook and then he passed. I miss him and keep in touch with his wife and daughter. Hmmm, lots of people have died in my 67 years. It's sad. Losing people is like collecting shadows. Some grow fainter over time, and others stay with you, sharp-edged, refusing to fade.

Looking through my picture albums, I found a picture of me in the cockpit of a commercial plane on a pilot's lap, pre-911, obviously. Did I mention I was a flirt? That's being kind, an understatement.

I applied for a gig as a PA when they were gearing up to make *Hills Have Eyes II*. Wes Craven made the original Hills in 1977 and wrote this sequel and planned to direct it as well. I decided to leave WMA since shooting films was more exciting. I was still living in North Hollywood and commuting to Hollywood for interviews and auditions.

It was there that I met Barry, one of the producers, and we started dating after I was hired. He was a nice Jewish guy, though not devout—just like me. Being Jewish meant it is in your DNA, and if you were a "good" Jew, you would go to temple, celebrate the high holidays, etc.

Mom was happy to hear that we were dating. Back in the day, perhaps even now, most Jewish mothers wanted their daughters to marry a Jewish doctor. If he wasn't a doctor, being Jewish was almost good enough.

As a PA on *Hills II*, my first assignment was to follow an old school bus to the desert, where it would be blown up at the end of the film. Crawling along at 35 miles per hour was torture for a NY driver like me—slow just isn't my jam (style).

Then during shooting, at the end of the day, I took the dailies (footage shot each day) to the lab in Hollywood. When we wrapped (finished shooting), we had the wrap party at the Grotto at Two Bunch Palms, a place steeped in history, where Al Capone once spent time. There was even a lookout tower, which was incredibly cool.

After we finished Hills II, Barry took me to Maui, and we went scuba diving. I discovered I was an island child the minute I stepped off the plane. We went to Acapulco and parasailed. We rode horses on the beach. We went water skiing.

He water skied; I fell down a lot. We went to Tahoe and snow skied. He skied; I fell down a lot (on the bunny slope!)

Barry had a sweet bungalow in Studio City. He made a lot of money, which was attractive to me since I disliked being poor. I still felt the need to be taken care of so I could pursue my dreams. He asked me to move in, and I accepted. He had many producer and director friends so we socialized a lot.

There was a LOT of cocaine. We both used it, but I think I used it more. I cooked while I was buzzed, which was probably 80 percent of my waking life.

Cooking became my ritual, my distraction, my proof that I had it together. Even when I didn't. I was buzzing and floating through life just enough to feel functional, never enough to feel whole.

I wanted to impress Barry's cronies with elaborate Thai meals that took me three days to shop for, cook, and make. The night they all came over for dinner, I passed out before they got there from exhaustion and depression. Nowadays, I think it's called imposter syndrome.

Barry and I went to visit Yui in Thailand. We went to Phuket and a bunch of other places. My very generous and kind friend Yui gave me the most exquisite emerald earrings. After she gave them to me, we all went to a bathhouse for massage. I was told to take off my jewelry, and like an idiot, I did. Someone stole the earrings. A hefty price to pay for a massage.

After that, Barry and I met Yui in Mexico. My very generous friend brought me an exquisite diamond pinky ring. It fell off while we were boating. Apparently, one of the crew saw it happen and grabbed it. When we got back to the hotel, he tried to hold it hostage for ransom. The concierge made him give it back. That was special, I must say!

We had a backward birthday party for Barry. All the women dressed as men, and all the men dressed as women. I had a cake made with a picture of him with boobs and me with a penis and chest hair on it.

1986

Barry's house in Studio City was right down the street from one of the stars of *Cagney and Lacey*. That's how I met Rob, my next "crush," and was again a cheater. Rob drove for one of the stars. You'd think I would have learned my lesson by this time. Nope. We had an affair. Fun fact? We used to call her show Gag Me and Rape Me. Rob did coke too, but back then, it seemed like nearly everyone was into it. He was also very attractive, with prematurely gray hair.

Barry got off the white powder, but try as I might, I couldn't. Quitting should have been easy—just stop, just walk away. But addiction isn't logic. It's a whisper in your brain that tells you you're better with it, that you need it, that life without it is worse than life drowning in it.

It took me losing him and the adorable home in Studio City to get me to finally quit. Barry had his attorney write a letter giving me $5,000 as a thank-you for my years of service. Barry's next girlfriend was named Sheri Smith, spelled just like I spell it! What are the odds?

I visited Yui again in Thailand, thanks to her kindness and generosity, as I couldn't afford the flight on my own. Once again, I had a fabulous time. I ended up meeting a great guy from Scandinavia, and we spent time together. A few weeks after I returned home, I received a stunning 24-karat gold necklace of two butterflies. He wrote that he had it made for me. It was such a thoughtful and extravagant gift, especially considering we would probably never see each other again. I was deeply touched and wore it constantly, never taking it off.

1987-1988

I was still auditioning for parts—film, TV, commercials, or whatever was listed in the *Hollywood Reporter*, which is how you found out about them. Auditions in LA were few and far between, unlike in NY, where you could "pound the pavement," as we used to say. In New York, I had an agent who sent me to auditions. In LA, I didn't have an agent. Since I was meeting with producers and directors who were hiring not only actors but also production staff, I started working for various producers in whatever capacity they needed, since I had skills and qualifications. This was akin to acting jobs since the gigs were for the shooting schedule, anywhere from four to eight weeks. I even preferred it since it wasn't about my looks or acting ability as much as my brain and typing. I'm eternally grateful to my Mom for strongly encouraging me to take typing in the '70s when I went to live with Nat.

When these production gigs ended, I worked at MGM, Warner Brothers, and then Telepictures as an executive assistant. At MGM, I worked for Jake. Flash forward to 2020, when I searched for him on LinkedIn. I asked him to connect. It's a thing I do—I have over 6,000 connections. I messaged him: "I doubt you re- member me, but I worked for you in 1988 at MGM. OMG, you haven't aged at ALL. Ok to connect?" He messaged back: "I have aged greatly! But I do remember you well. You were the very cute one who made me uncomfortable with your inappropriateness! Fortunately, it was long before today's #MeToo era. Nonetheless, it was a good thing that I'm such a nerd. Be happy to connect. Hope you're well." Poor guy. But he had the class to respond and was truthful. That says a lot about a person's character, in my opinion. I left MGM. Why? Oh, I remember, it was corporate, that's right. I was a nonconformist.

One of my bosses nurtured my entrepreneurial spirit, often entrusting me with personal errands in addition to my office duties, which I adored. I took his car in for service, looked after his Malibu bungalow when he traveled, and even organized a beach party complete with food and entertainment—my first taste of event coordination. In hindsight, I'll always be grateful for his support. I just wish I had pursued that career path back then! I accomplished his errands so well that he suggested I start a company doing errands for Hollywood execs. It sounded like a great idea, so I did. I started a company called Executive Express, Your Personal Runaround. I was covered on the front page of the *LA Times* business section and that led to articles in *Working Woman* and *Big Valley* magazines. They are all in my book *When We Wrote Letters, The Eighties.*

Pam Dauber, an actress and Mark Harmon's wife, saw the article in *The Times* and had a script written loosely based on my company called "This Wife For Hire." At about the same time, I thought I would like to train dogs, and I could market both of these entities. I printed up a flier for Puppy Love, Obedience, and Protection Training. My tagline was: if you have a dog, you need a dog trainer. I offered courses in basic obedience, advanced off-leash, and personal protection and gave a lifetime guarantee. I never got even one client, which, looking back, was probably a good thing.

1989

My company wasn't generating enough income. It was during this period of financial uncertainty that I stumbled upon the world of MLM (multi level marketing). Specifically with a company called NuSkin, that developed and distributed personal care products and nutritional supplements. Some of my clients even regrew hair using one of the products. The skincare line was an added bonus, especially with the discounted rates. I organized product demonstrations at senior living communities since wrinkles were plentiful. We got great results putting the product on one half of a wrinkled face. I excelled and quickly rose through the ranks of distributorship.

I did so well that a start-up offering a diet patch headhunted me. They wanted me to join their corporate team to help launch the company—no selling involved, just overseeing operations. But once inside, I quickly realized the company was taking advantage of thousands of people. The patch had no proprietary formula and was essentially a scam. I watched as they took money for a product that didn't exist beyond someone's imagination. Lose weight by putting on a patch? Unbelievable, yet that's exactly what people who wanted to lose weight wanted to believe. Lose weight by slapping on a sticker. The logic was nonexistent, but desperation doesn't ask for logic. It just reaches for the next magic trick.

As the company was circling the drain, they decided to launch by having lunch for 1,500 of their members from all around the country. The bosses gave me the business card of a caterer (J's) and told me to contract with him. I made an appointment for him to come in to discuss it. He came to meet me with one of the first mobile phones ever on his shoulder. It must've weighed 15 pounds. Was I impressed? I'm not sure. I had never seen one before and imagined it would be great to get charged a fortune to be able to make calls when the fancy struck.

Lunch for the crowd was to be all-you-can-eat ribs and chicken. J was only going to charge eight dollars per guest including drinks and cookies. I grabbed his contract, signed it, and then yelled at him for not charging enough. I made sure he knew to get the full amount before he brought the lunch. Thankfully for him, he took my advice and didn't get stiffed like many other vendors did. When the company went belly up shortly thereafter, I was left without a job and an occupation, wondering WHAT THE HELL to do with my life—AGAIN. Every time I thought I'd found my path, the ground crumbled beneath me. AGAIN. Reinventing myself was becoming a full-time job, and honestly? I was exhausted.

I got depressed and started drinking more and more to numb myself and self-medicate. One night, I was drunk off my ass, and I got stopped by the police. I should've been arrested and thrown in jail. That was in the '80s, and alarmingly, shockingly, they let me go because I was only a few miles from my house. How I got home and parked in the garage is another mystery. When I woke up the next day, I ran out to see if my car was there and in one piece and was relieved to see it was. How did I get to be this person? I'd always drank, smoked cigs and pot, and used coke, but things were getting worse.

I was still living in North Hollywood and driving my little minivan down to Irvine every day to work for that MLM company and discovered I liked the OC (Orange County). My relationship with Rob was going nowhere. I knew we were at the end and had to break up. He moved out.

I had a brilliant idea to approach J for a job. I presented myself to him at his kitchen. He had transformed an empty 3,000-square-foot warehouse into a fully functional kitchen. He was a talented carpenter and construction person and did it all — walls, electrical, everything. I asked for a tour and a job. I realized it was my first time inside a walk-in fridge and freezer. I fell madly in love. With the kitchen, not J. He was married. I think I finally learned my lesson about the sanctity of marriage.

He told me he was going through bankruptcy and couldn't hire anyone. That should have been my first hint. I told him he didn't have to pay me to come in every day and try to sell events. I would take a percentage or a commission only if I sold something. He accepted my offer. Most days, we'd work late into the night. I made a proposal for an AIDS fundraiser and submitted it to Elizabeth Taylor. She passed it along to Elizabeth Glaser's pediatric AIDS Foundation, but they never bothered to respond. A year later, I opened *People* magazine and saw they had a successful fundraiser event in Beverly Hills based on all the ideas I'd proposed. Who needed a nobody caterer in Orange County? I was gratified to know that my idea was a good one.

Driving from the San Fernando Valley every day was challenging, to say the least. I drove a minivan and tried to remember to take things, such as a change of clothes and toiletries, and had enough room to schlep everything, but the car was always a mess with my belongings strewn everywhere. J built cabinets in the car for me. That was special.

Long story short, in no particular order: we had sex while he was separated but still married, which didn't seem like a big thing to me, but it was a major thing in the LDS church. So, it was decided that he and his soon-to-be ex, Lynette, would drive together to Vegas for a "quickie" divorce. He got excommunicated from the Mormon church because we had sex before he was actually divorced. Later, he crawled his way back into the church's good graces and was reinstated. He made me take missionary lessons and wanted me to join the church. I did.

Then the missionaries told me I had to get baptized. I told them I'd already been baptized. (Actually a Jewish girlfriend grabbed me one day and took me to church and we were both baptized before I met J. My mom didn't speak to me for years.) I was told, "You weren't baptized with authority," according to the Mormons, so I had to do it again.

He owned a small plane, and our first "official" date after the divorce was to visit my parents in Vegas. He let me take the controls and "fly" for a bit. Unfortunately, not long after that, he had to hand over the plane to Joe, his attorney, for fees he owed him for the bankruptcy.

We decided to get married. Would I NEVER stop making HORRIBLE decisions?

At this point, I had to wonder—was I cursed? Did I have some karmic debt to pay? Or was I just really, really bad at picking men?

We picked the date of January 19, 1989, to get married since my birthday is March 19, hoping it would make it an easy date for us to remember.

We moved into the house he shared with Lynette to fix it up and sell it. During the move from North Hollywood to Orange County, we were transporting my two antique stained-glass windows. Unfortunately, he accidentally put his knee through one of them. What was once valued at nearly $1,000 was now almost worthless due to the damage. I was heartbroken.

When you file for Chapter 7 bankruptcy, the trustee seizes your assets, which happened to J. They locked up the kitchen, so he couldn't get in. I should have seen the flashing neon signs warning me away. But I was already in too deep—financially, emotionally, stupidly.

The whole point of filing was to "start over." We needed to buy the assets from the bankruptcy court to resume catering. Neither of our parents trusted him with a nickel because he was horrible at managing money. They each lent ME $10,000. I bought the assets from the bankruptcy court. We named the new entity Gourmet

Catering. PS: our parents got their money back pronto.

On July 14, 1989, we started a journal. It was VERY enlightening. I photocopied it, released it, and called it *Journal of a Bipolar Marriage.* (WHY DIDN'T I RUN AWAY?) I came to discover years later that I was bullied and allowed it. Huh? I always considered myself to be a bright person. WHY on earth did I allow it? Making matters worse, he had a condition called Peyronie's disease, which causes the penis to curve during erections due to internal scar tissue. While it didn't bother him, it was painful for me when we had sex.

I am an enigma, a paradox, a walking contradiction. Some might call me weird, but I prefer to think of it as my endearing eccentricities, unique characteristics, and lovable oddities—my one-of-a-kind traits. And let's not forget: I'm just ahead of my time.

A few examples:

1. I will eat a bowlful of food I don't care for IF it's jam-packed with nutrition

and health, *even* if it tastes horrible. But if it has garlic, turmeric, ginger, spicy peppers, and everything else that protects and nourishes my body temple, I'm in. Nutritional yeast, flax, tons of EVOO. When I make oatmeal? It can't be just any oatmeal; it must be steel-cut oatmeal. I add a few tablespoons of Cream of Wheat for extra iron, almond and/or nut butter, elderberry syrup, ghee, or grass-fed butter. Can I get any more nutrients in it? Maybe, but I don't think so. It is ironic to me that I do this NOW after a life of self-abuse. Smoking cigarettes in my teens, then pot, and drinking beer for lunch in my 20s and beyond. Trying LSD and Psilocybin. Then, on to abusing cocaine, pain meds, uppers, downers, and everything in between. Actually, I marvel that I am still alive.

2. I've saved EVERYTHING from my life. I kept every single letter,

postcard, greeting card, calendar, appointment book, and some paystubs from my first job(s) in the '70s. I even saved a month of birth control pills. Huh? Probably after I got "fixed" and didn't need them anymore. I started filling up a Rubbermaid trunk. If I loved a T-shirt a lot, I cut out the front, the "saying," and threw it in. Perhaps I thought one day I'd make a quilt. I don't sew, but a dear friend (shoutout to Janet) makes quilts. Nah, that won't happen. I've schlepped the trunk around with me all these years, starting in the 60's. From NY to Mexico and back, from NY to Vegas and back. From NY to California, to Hawaii, and back.

3. No matter how many times I lose the lottery, I know one day I WILL win, so I keep throwing my hard-earned money at it. Doesn't everybody? I truly believe I will win the lottery one day. Odds be

damned. Delusion? Optimism? Who cares? Some people collect stamps, I collect hope.

4. Ahead of my time? There are NOW news pieces about things I've been doing for years. You don't need supplements. YES, supplements are good! Eggs are good; eggs are bad. I guess you must follow the science, and I do. You were supposed to eat like a king for breakfast when you awoke, a prince for lunch, and a pauper for dinner. I never did that, preferring to starve until I couldn't take it anymore. Now, intermittent fasting is WONDERFUL for you, meaning you shouldn't eat for at least twelve hours or more after your meal the night before. I've always done that, and I imagine I always will do it.

5. I've been taking supplements since the '70s. When I had a full hysterectomy in 1998, I made a recovery program for myself. I took a little baggie of

supplements and vitamins morning, afternoon, and night. I never got one hot flash. Thank you, black cohosh et al. Now, in the 2020s, doctors are acknowledging we should ALL take supplements, especially as we age. Yep.

6. Drinking coffee is good for you; drinking it is bad for you. Now, they are telling us that one to two cups a day is actually good for you. I always knew that or loved it so much that I closed my ears to any negativity. Keep coffee (beans) in the fridge or freezer; then, there is no need to … just keep it in a cabinet.

7. Everyone asks: "How did you get the URL GourmetCatering.com?" I saw the internet coming down the pike and hopped on.

8. I keep disposable gloves in my car. When I find a dead animal (pet cat or dog, raccoon, or skunk), I take it out of

the road. If it's a pet, I look for a tag to contact the owner. Then, I call the authorities to pick up the carcass.

9. Global Warming. Now, folks are figuring out they need to recycle and be mindful of our planet. Catch up people. Zero Waste movement; uh, yes, please.

10. Buy Nothing. FB has a page for each neighborhood. Recycle, reuse, and save the planet. I found out about it and jumped on. Then our local TV news station, ABC7, did a piece on it.

11. Wait 30 minutes after eating before swimming. The science now says that is a bunch of hooey (no need). And as a daily swimmer, I agree and actually prefer to have something beforehand.

12. When #CovidCrap started and they said "Social Distancing," I kept screaming PHYSICAL distancing. Turns out I was right.

More Examples of "Weird":

1. I give everybody a lovey-dovey name, as I call it. A lot of people call it a nickname. No matter what you call it. That is just me. Even a simple name like Mark? I call my friend Marky.

2. I abbreviate. Examples: FB (Facebook), SC (sweetheart cottage), CH (carriage house), CIH (Castle in Hawaii), and CF (chocolate fountain). I have no good reason, excuse, or explanation.

3. I have eco-anxiety and while it is not classified as a clinical disorder, it is recognized as a natural response to the real and overwhelming challenges of the current environmental situation. I often stress over how to dispose of things. Take recycling, for example. Cans often have residue—should I rinse them out and waste water, or dispose of them as is and risk contaminating the recycling? These small,

everyday decisions become sources of worry.

4. I talk to myself. Doesn't everyone? Sometimes, myself talks back. It's kind of comforting that someone's listening. It's a full conversation. Sometimes questions, answers, arguments. The best part? I always win.

5. I dislike feeling out of touch, especially with language that is constantly changing. I offered someone something, and she said, "I'm down," I had to think and translate in my brain. Oh, that meant she wanted it. The kids today. I think George and I had the same issues back in the day. Love you, Dad! I finally get it now.

The '90s

This was a busy decade. I was obsessed with making Gourmet Catering a household name. We worked our tails off. The lion's share of the business was catering for nonprofits with a slim profit margin—high schools, churches, etc.—with a few weddings and corporate events thrown in. I wanted to do more upscale events. There was a bit of a learning curve, but it was not brain surgery.

I learned about an annual convention called Catersource. Mike Roman was a visionary entrepreneur who was passionate about food service and recognized a glaring gap in the industry: the lack of a dedicated platform for caterers to learn, network, and grow. He founded the convention to help caterers expand their knowledge. I credit my attendance with bringing our gross to over one million.

It was there I met PP and fell in love—the moment she took the stage, I was mesmerized. It was a full-blown girl crush, the first since summer camp, but this wasn't just admiration. She was the caterer I longed to become British style. A powerhouse executing the kind of upscale events I aspired to do. I sat rapt in the audience, furiously taking notes (this was the stone age, after all) as she shared her vast knowledge.

Around this time, we were asked if we would sponsor an exchange student. I didn't have to think twice. He turned out to be the son I never had—and a rocket scientist to boot! He worked picnics for us during the summer and after the year was up, he went back to Spain and wrote faithfully. He was a brilliant and kind human, and we were lucky to have him.

J's mom, Carol, was our bookkeeper; his sister sold events for us, and we had a guy who sold nonprofit events. Then, we hired another man who sold corporate events. He ended up having a heart attack in the walk-in, which was scary.

Carol had a ranch in the desert, which was about 100 miles from where we lived. It was the high desert, and it generally gets much hotter in the summer and much colder in the winter than LA. She was married to Tim, her fifth marriage. She bred horses and had four or more mares at any one time and two studs. The whole family, including J's half-brother Stan, his wife, and four kids, liked to spend weekends there when there were no catering jobs. We played board games, card games and rode.

There was a stable near our house in Fullerton. It wasn't a building like a typical stable; it had about twenty covered stalls. The owners of the horses put all their gear in storage sheds in front of the stalls. I'd sneak over there whenever I needed some horsey love, recalling happy times at Camp Wishe. One day, the lady who owned it and knew about Carol's ranch told me a stall had become available. She suggested I lease a horse. Huh? She explained that leasing a horse is like renting. You're on the hook for food and board, but the payoff? You get to ride whenever you want. It was the best of both worlds—all the perks of having a horse without the commitment of owning one.

It worked out perfectly since Carol was happy to have her mares get individual attention as they languished in stalls at the ranch. Lady, Flame, and Aldezar were among my favorites. She'd get one of them pregnant, then let me lease the mom-to-be. The month before she was ready to drop the foal, I would trailer her back to the ranch.

Horses have an unspoken agreement with the universe: they almost always give birth under the cover of night, long after the world has quieted. I have hours of footage—mares shifting anxiously, the first tremors of labor, the final push, and that breathtaking moment when a new life takes its first unsteady breaths, then steps.

The day the mare indicated she was going to give birth, Carol would call me, and I would pack a chaise lounge, a lantern, and a video camera and race out to the desert after rush hour traffic subsided. Sitting there in the dim glow of my lantern, watching a tiny, slick foal struggle to stand on wobbly legs, I always felt an overwhelming mix of emotions. Awe. Joy. The kind of deep, soul-level peace that comes from witnessing life begin.

Irvine Meadows was a popular concert venue in Orange County, and we scored exclusive rights to cater. Sweet! We catered to every popular musician, band, and group at the time. When Michael Jackson came to do a show, he brought Bubbles, his chimp. That would have been fine had he not brought the animal through the catering buffet line. Luckily, the Department of Health didn't inspect events on Saturday.

The stable's location at a busy intersection meant every trail ride began with a tense journey navigating several blocks of concrete and asphalt streets, dealing with traffic and noise, before finally reaching the trail. If we kept it slow, we were usually okay. But the week before the Moody Blues concert—one of my top five bands ever—disaster struck. Some idiot honked their horn, spooking Lady, my mare at the time. She bolted, slipped, and we went down hard. She tore the flap of skin (flank) between the leg bones and the rib bones. When I hit the ground I twisted my knee. The next thing I knew, I was in a bulky knee brace just days before the Moody Blues concert. Talk about bad timing!

After serving the buffet, when it came time to watch the show, a kindhearted roadie saw me and took pity. He hoisted me up to the side of the stage, giving me a bird's-eye view where I wouldn't get jostled.

All of our salespeople, myself included, had a computer. While I mostly worked from home, the rest of the team worked from the kitchen. We all needed to stay aligned on what the others were proposing, so we all needed access to the same information to ensure consistency. J read a thick, dry, boring book on computer programming. When he was done, he had developed a computer program for catering. We were all impressed. One December, from the first until the twenty-fourth, we had as many as fifteen events in one day. We were so organized because of the program that most went off without a hitch.

Joe, J's attorney, found and married a woman who lived just a couple of miles from him in Fullerton, only about five miles from the kitchen in Buena Park. He planned to put his house on the market—cue the screeching brakes. We asked if we could buy it. Knowing how financially strapped we were since the bankruptcy, Joe knew we wouldn't qualify for a traditional bank loan. He agreed to sell it to us and carry the loan himself, meaning we would make payments directly to him instead of a bank. And since we couldn't afford to buy furnishings, and since his new wife had a complete domicile, we told him, "Just pack your clothes and leave everything else." And that's exactly what he did.

We became the proud owners of the most amazing three-bedroom, two-bath home with a pool, a gorgeous kitchen, a huge rec room, a living room, and an atrium. The backyard had a rose garden, which I promptly ripped out to plant a mango tree. I also added berries, bananas, and plumeria—determined to recreate a little slice of Hawaii in our backyard, island style. Joe handled all the finances, doing the calculations on a spreadsheet by hand—crazy. We paid him a minimum of $2,000 a month and more if we did well, during the busy summer picnic season and December peak season with holiday events.

J bought a motorcycle. I bought a million-dollar life insurance policy on him. One of us was making smart choices.

A woman rear-ended him, and he dropped the motorcycle and slid on the asphalt, resulting in a trip to the hospital for road rash (severe skin abrasion). J sold the bike.

I canceled the policy.

1991

We were putting together a great team of dishwashers, cooks, waitstaff and salespeople. We were growing and growing. I wrote "Team Guidelines." This was to create a clear set of standards for housekeeping and operations and help ensure everyone was on the same page, fostering consistency and teamwork as we scaled up. People would ask, "Where is such and such ... ?" and we had a saying: "If it were up your butt, you'd know."

One of our dishwashers came all the way from Santa Ana to wash dishes. He was excellent at his job and very conscientious. We loved him! When he didn't come in one day in June, we were concerned, and it turned out he shot someone after drinking and while playing cards. It was a pity. He was a good man. We all make mistakes, but this landed him in jail after the guy died from the gunshot wound.

Newsletters to and from your family were popular in the nineties, saving time not writing to everyone individually. I wrote one "to everyone":

Dear Everyone:

I'm writing to all my friends and loved ones to bring you "up to speed" on my life. I've had no time to call, write, or have a life for the past month. Why? Where shall I start? In September business was grim. Catering, like every other industry, has been getting slower by the minute. No one is spending any money these days. Recession? Depression?

J saw an ad in a food publication. A man, Shane, wanted to sell a TV and movie catering company in North Hollywood. Buying a company couldn't have been further from our minds, especially with our cash flow situation being so poor at the time. We were barely staying afloat, so acquiring a business just wasn't on the radar.

But for some reason, we were compelled to drive up to the valley for a "look-see." It's about a 45-minute drive without traffic. To make a long story short, I asked him what church he and his family went to. Of course, it was the LDS church, and suddenly, all the walls and barriers melted.

It turns out Shane had been "screwed" twice, and he was now at the same point we were three years ago—about to declare bankruptcy. The bottom line? We decided to join forces. He's a super salesperson and took his business to $1.4

million, working out of a small kitchen with four catering trucks for films, not to be confused with the roach coaches that sell food to companies at lunchtime.

His client list was to die for. He catered some of the most popular TV shows at the time: Empty Nest, Night Court, Murphy Brown, and Designing Women, plus a bunch of films. He was embezzled for about $20-$25K and had been mismanaged. He had what we didn't—sales. We had what he didn't—a huge kitchen and a terrific staff.

At the beginning of October, our chef notified us that he was leaving. He didn't even have the courtesy to give two weeks' notice. Right about this time, we learned that the jerk J hired to do our books was an incompetent a*hole, to be kind. He made a $1,000 deposit and recorded it as $10,000. So now we were overdrawn $9,000.

Our director of operations was discontented because we were buying a house and he was renting an apartment. So J gave him 10% of our stock, hoping that would placate him. It didn't. He signed a "noncompete" contract, and despite that, he and the chef decided to start their own company. They came into the office in the middle of the night, dumped our computer data onto discs, and started contacting our clients. Most of the clients were loyal and called me and told me they had been contacted. They even sent me the menus and marketing literature that they were sent! Which was MY literature. Literature that I had carefully crafted over the past three years. They weren't just poaching our clients—they were using my own words to do so. My carefully crafted menus, my marketing, my blood, sweat, and years of work repackaged as their own.

This sounds like a disaster, but it was actually a blessing. At the time, it felt like a sucker punch to the gut. Like being stabbed in the back, then handed the knife so I could twist it myself.

Shane relocated his catering business to our warehouse, bringing his chef with him, and we caught those turncoats snooping over the fence as he was moving in. Good. I hope they're eating their hearts out. They deserved each other. We took over the warehouse next to the two we already had, which gave us an additional 2,800 square feet. We had to build a new 20' x 30' walk-in fridge.

J and I work twelve to twenty hours a day, six to seven days a week. Shelly, our new chef, has been with Shane for years and is a superwoman besides super chef! She works over forty hours a week while raising two small sons.

Now that you're totally bored to tears with the trials and tribulations of being an entrepreneur, see the enclosed copy of an article on bartering … guess who's in it? With a color picture! I'm now trying for another one in *Entrepreneurial Woman*. Wish me luck.

I just read *Scarlett*, the sequel to Margaret Mitchell's *Gone with the Wind*. It's my only reprieve from work and sleep: 800 pages, and I adored it! *Gone with the Wind* was my favorite book and movie ever.

The thing that is keeping me going is waiting for December 24. Why? I'm getting on a plane and will be in Hawaii five hours later. I booked this trip four months ago and have already made lists about what I will take and what I want to do when I get there. I'll only be gone for one week—we get back the day before New Year's just in case any parties book and we have to work.

I'd love to hear from you. Love you all, hope you are all ok. Write. Send pics.

PS: The partnership with Shane didn't work out, perhaps due to the challenges posed by him having to commute from the Valley to our kitchen in Orange County. Additionally, he and J often couldn't see eye to eye; both were strong-willed individuals who wanted to be the boss, leading to frequent power struggles and disagreements.

1992

February 27

Mom and George were in LA for their business. We had plans to get together. Suddenly I got a frantic call from Mom, who told me to meet her at Good Samaritan Hospital. George had suffered a heart attack. I dropped everything and flew there in a panic.

When I arrived, they were assessing his condition. Then he had another heart attack. Mom and I stood there helplessly, watching as they worked on him, trying to revive him, performing CPR for what felt like an eternity. He started swelling from all the drugs they were pumping into him by IV (intravenous, "within or into a vein.") Which didn't seem to do anything for him. Finally, I told them to stop. Mom begged them not to stop. He wasn't supposed to die. Not now. Not ever.

He was not responding to all the meds or the CPR. I had to accept that his life couldn't continue. It was his time. She could not accept it. He passed away right in front of us. Watching her crumble next to his hospital bed, I felt utterly helpless.

She returned to Vegas to sit shiva, the traditional Jewish mourning period, with her friends gathered around to offer support and comfort. I had to stay in LA because of work obligations, and though it pained me not to be by her side, she understood the demands I faced. Despite the physical distance, I stayed connected the only way I could. I called her twice a day. Those brief moments over the phone were my way of reassuring her that even though I couldn't be there in person, my heart was with her. Every call ended with "I love you," a simple reminder that my love bridged the miles between us.

1993

I found out Mom connected with an old friend, Don Cherry. They say that, especially as you grow older, if someone passes away, it's probable, perhaps inevitable, that you will marry a dear friend rather than date.

Don was an American pop music singer, big band singer, and celebrity golfer. More importantly, he was the person Mom needed after losing George. He was born in Texas and had made many albums, published a biography,

Cherry's Jubilee, and was a dear friend of Willie Nelson. He played golf with the likes of Arnold Palmer and won green jackets in the Masters Tournaments. He had been married three times before marrying Mom. He was a teetotaler and had never smoked. Mom had smoked but quit. They made the perfect couple. He moved into Mom's house in Vegas, and they lived happily ever after. Watching them together, I felt relief. She wasn't just surviving. She was living again.

As we were growing Gourmet Catering, we were building out our fleet of trucks. We named them all. Our Utilimaster Johnny Cab was Johnny. My dad helped us buy a truck, so we named it George, but we called him Geo. Another one, a high cube with a lift gate, was BOT (big old truck).

All the trucks required regular maintenance, and there was a tire shop just a mile down the road with an excellent reputation. The last thing we could afford was a truck breaking down on the way to an event. That would have been a disaster. J brought a few vehicles there and we realized we'd struck gold with the owner, Jeff. He was more than honest; he treated every vehicle like it was his own. Before long, Jeff wasn't just our trusted mechanic—he became a friend, someone we could rely on.

Life has a way of bringing kindred spirits together, I guess. While Jeff was struggling through a nightmarish divorce with his wife, who had mental health challenges, I was unknowingly soon to be on the brink of my own marital meltdown. His son inherited his mom's mental health struggles, a "gift" no parent wants to pass on. Jeff was a caregiver and very kind.

I spent a lot of time scouting locations for events, particularly parks for corporate picnics, which were always in high demand. Securing the right spot was crucial for booking large-scale events. One of our competitors, flush with cash, had the foresight to buy up many prime locations.

One day, as I was heading to check out a Regional Park to the east of us, I noticed a large sign in an unexpected area. Something compelled me to investigate, though I wasn't sure why. I just trusted my gut. Long story short, I found the people who oversaw the property. It was about eight acres and would be able to hold thousands of guests. We made a deal to improve it and utilize it for company picnics. We named it Wildcatters. This park would ultimately be instrumental in raising our gross revenue. The Brea Chamber wrote about it in their newsletter. Unfortunately, they didn't get our name right. They called us Gourmet Caterers. Oh well.

When we first started doing large company picnics, we needed to include supervised picnic game packages with prizes for the children. I developed a program of games and competitions. They included candy on a spoon, cup of water on the head, tug-of-war, bubble gum blowing, egg toss, pie eating, bingo, and others. In the beginning I ran the games with the help of a script so I wouldn't forget anything. We gave prizes to the winners and my favorite part was shopping for the prizes.

To take a break from the demands of catering, I volunteered at the Wildlife Waystation. I was assigned chimp enrichment tasks. Around the same time, my passion for nontraditional pets led me to adopt two minks—unaware that they were a male and female pair—which led to an unexpected litter. Unfortunately, one of the babies fell from the cage, which made me decide to rehome them. I also had chinchillas, drawn to anything furry that piqued my interest, but this time I ensured they were the same sex to avoid surprises.

For a few years, I had issues with what I thought was my stomach. Once a year, I'd have acute attacks of incredible, intense pain. I self-diagnosed it as a stomach problem.

When I finally went to the ER, they said go to a GYN. Huh? I ended up having a total hysterectomy. They took it all—ovaries, uterus—and my libido with it. It was probably the best thing that ever happened to me. More proof that I am weird? I asked the doctor for my organs. I didn't get them, but they did give me Polaroids of them.

The director of operations at Irvine Meadows decided to go catering in-house so we lost the account. Major bummer. Fortunately, we secured an account catering Hoag Hospital's monthly midnight meal, which replaced some of the lost income, as did the publicity we garnered here and there.

1994

In June, J and I finally began seeing a marriage counselor, a decision that had taken months—if not years—of tension, arguments, and failed attempts to fix things on our own. We were both at a breaking point, uncertain if the relationship could even be saved, but neither of us was willing to give up entirely. Sitting in that small, neutral room with tissues on the table and a clock ticking softly in the background, I had no idea what to expect. I wasn't sure if we would walk out closer together or farther apart. I only knew that if we didn't try, the damage would be irreparable.

The early sessions were difficult. We were both guarded, defensive, and reluctant to fully open up. But slowly, under the gentle guidance of the counselor, we began to peel back layers we had both carefully built over the years. Then, one afternoon, everything changed. It started as a seemingly ordinary session, but as we delved deeper into a particular argument, J became un-characteristically quiet. His eyes shifted down-ward; his hands clenched in his lap. When he finally spoke, his voice was low and halting, as if each word carried the weight of years of silence.

"I was raped when I was a child," he said. The room went completely still. My breath caught in my throat, and for a moment, I wasn't sure I had heard him correctly. And for a split second, I wished I hadn't heard him at all. What do you do or say after a revelation like that? I wanted to hold him, to somehow erase the pain, but I knew some wounds never fully heal.

But then he continued, his words spilling out in a way that felt both urgent and hesitant as if part of him was desperate to let the truth out while another part wanted to keep it buried. He went on to describe growing up in a violent home, a place where fear and pain were constants by the stepfathers his mom married, where safety was a luxury he never experienced. I was stunned. My mind raced as I tried to reconcile this revelation with the man I thought I knew. It was as if a light had been shone on years of confusion, illuminating things that had always been just out of my understanding. The anger, the defensiveness, the emotional distance—it all suddenly made sense. For years, I had taken his behavior personally, interpreting it as rejection, indifference, or even malice. But now, I saw it for what it was: a survival mechanism, a way of coping with pain so deep that it had shaped every part of him.

As the weight of his words settled over the room, I felt a flood of emotions I couldn't begin to untangle. Compassion came first—a deep, aching sorrow for the little boy who had endured such unimaginable trauma. Then came guilt, sharp and unrelenting. How many times had I lashed out at him in frustration, not understanding the deeper wounds beneath his actions? How many arguments could have been avoided if I had known the truth? But there was also anger—not at him, but at the people and circumstances that had hurt him so profoundly. Anger at the injustice of it all, that someone I loved had been forced to carry such a heavy burden for so long.

What do you do with a revelation like that? How do you support someone through a pain so vast, so ingrained, that it has become part of their very being? I wanted to fix it, to take the pain away, but I knew I couldn't. The counselor tried to guide us through the conversation, but my mind kept returning to one overwhelming thought: How had J carried this all alone for so long? And what did it mean for us now?

As usual we threw ourselves into our business and work.In November, we were featured in the *Orange County Register* for a surprise wedding we catered. It was fun, and the publicity? Priceless.

1996

We had the incredible opportunity to cater a fundraiser for the Wildlife Waystation at Mayor Riordan's beautiful home in Brentwood. This event stands out as the highlight of my career. The legendary Betty White graced us with her presence, and we were all thrilled to see a tiger and other exotic animals up close. To top it all off, we featured an ice sculpture that added a touch of elegance. We used our copper chafers, and I designed a snake of salmon, cream cheese, capers, lemon wedges, and caviar with black olive eyes that slithered across granite blocks. It was spectacular if I say so myself—and I do.

1997

I was obsessed with getting more and more sales and determined to get us to $1 million! I always believed my self-worth was attached to my income. Doesn't everyone? Well, drum roll, please … in 1998, we broke a million.

1998

J's half-brother, Stan, was also a caterer, and basically, a competitor, which seemed crazy to me. I suggested that we join forces. Again, will I NEVER learn?

In just a few years, he and his sibling severely mismanaged a thriving catering business that headed us towards our demise. I learned there were serious ethical breaches, including mis-use of company funds and deception with our salespeople and clients. At one point, a payment meant for the business was diverted, and the company name was even manipulated to deposit the check elsewhere. It was a betrayal of trust that left me disillusioned and scrambling to repair the damage. Despite assurances to the salesperson that the funds, a deposit for an upcoming event, hadn't been received, the truth eventually came to light, leading to a complicated financial fallout.

1999

We were grateful to our clients and showed it.
One day I made an appointment with three of
our best clients and our top (female) salespersons
and told them to pack their swimsuits and towels
and be in front of their houses at a certain time. I
showed up in a limo with a few bottles of champagne. We went to Glen Ivy Hot Springs, we
called it Club Mud. Relaxing massages, soaking
in the jacuzzi, playing in the mud, swimming,

then mani-pedis (manicure-pedicure). It was heaven after all the hard work we had done.

Our vendor, Sysco, was grateful to us, and they showed it. We spent so much money with them that they rewarded us with a cruise to the Caribbean on Dawn Princess. I loved it. If you are a caterer, having great food cooked for you is a dream come true. The next year, they sent us on a cruise to Alaska. It was not my cup of tea. I dislike cold weather, and how many falling glaciers can a person watch? So, instead, we ate and ate and ate and ate. Did I mention we ate?

We ventured into catering craft services for movies. It was simple to provide the cast and crew with a table of snacks, drinks, and mini meals. We had sold our two roach coaches after Shane left. I missed being on a set.

Since I worked mainly from home, unbeknownst to me, there were serious operational issues brewing behind the scenes at the kitchen, including unpaid taxes as well as strained relations with our employees. The mounting tensions led to losses—both in finances, equipment and trust. At one point, valuable equipment went missing, a sign of just how disjointed the situation had become. $600 copper chafers walked out the back door. Our business partners had invested in equipment, but as financial troubles mounted and bankruptcy loomed, many assets mysteriously vanished.

By the time 2000 rolled around, our business, worth $3.5 million, had been reduced to near ruins. We had built a $3.5 million empire from nothing. And in what felt like the blink of an eye, it was nothing again. I was pressured into signing over the remnants of the business for a token (symbolic) sum. It was a bitter moment, as the business I'd worked so hard to build up was dismantled and picked apart.

By 1999, we had $150K in equity in our house. The agreement/sale had never been recorded in 1990 because J was paranoid that the powers that be would take the house since he was in bankruptcy.

The 2000s

It was the start of a new century. Everyone was anxious about the "Y2K bug" and the fear that it would cause computer glitches and disruptions to vital systems worldwide.In the end, nothing was disrupted.

J's mom died, I found myself wanting a divorce. J's mom's passing seemed to flip a switch in him. Grief turned into something darker. The man I had once trusted became unpredictable. One night, in a fit of rage, he hurled a dining room chair through the plate glass window, shards exploding like tiny daggers across the floor. I stood there, frozen. This wasn't just stress or frustration, this was something deeper, something I didn't know how to handle.

It escalated to the point where I had to file for a restraining order. He was supposed to stay away from me, and one day I walked into the kitchen and found him sitting at one of the desks as if nothing had happened. I called the police, and they arrested him. The court mandated he attend anger management classes, but despite completing them, nothing changed. His behavior remained exactly the same.

All that being said, he didn't get diagnosed with bipolar disorder until he went to jail years later. (Oops, spoiler alert.) In those days, we had no clue about bipolar. People didn't discuss mental health. Later, I found out it lays dormant in some people, and when stress and anxiety build—BOOM—out it comes.

We were circling the drain financially. J was mismanaging the business. Déjà vu. J's dad sent

$20,000 to help us out, and J intercepted the check and took the money. He also took our little Dolphin motorhome, shipped it to the Big Island and moved there. He left me in California to deal with the sinking ship.

When J left, I got ferrets to distract and entertain me. Ferrets are illegal in California. People who owned ferrets had a saying: "Not game—PETS!" You had to get them surreptitiously. I discovered one of my neighbors had one she wanted to rehome, so I adopted him. I didn't want him to be lonely, so I found another through the ferret grapevine. Two turned into three, and I decided I had enough. Their names were Bobo, Niko, and Rocky. I bought them a condo. It looked like a giant bird cage but was designed especially for ferrets, with ramps and levels to hang out on and hammocks for snoozing. I let them out in my bedroom to play and had my Sony camcorder handy because it was always a laugh riot. I put a litter box in the closet, just in case they needed one when they were roaming around, but they mostly missed and did their business on my carpet. It was hard to think about my life falling apart at the seams while I was caring for, and cleaning up, after them.

I discovered that J purchased a parcel of land on the Big Island in Kalapana Seaview for $8,000, with a friend. The lot was located near the lava flow, and they put it in his friend's name to conceal the fact that he had an asset.

A year later, he decided he was tired of living in poverty. He called me, asking if he could borrow $100—though with him, "borrow" usually meant "have." And, being the sucker that I am, I sent it to him. After that, he started writing me, urging me to come to Hawaii, apologizing and claiming we could heal together. He also mentioned the lot he'd bought, but said he would give it up because, according to him, we needed to own property together and rebuild our family.

2001

September 11

At 5 a.m., I was in bed watching the news. About 45 minutes into the broadcast, the first plane hit the North Tower in Manhattan. I sat glued to the news, watching in absolute horror for hours. Eventually, I felt steady enough to call J in Hawaii, where it was three hours earlier than California that September morning.

Some days later, Mom called to tell me Don's son Stephen was a casualty of the attacks in the North Tower. He left behind four sons, left without a father. A family shattered in an instant. The world felt different that day, heavier. It was a reminder that life could change in a heartbeat.

The terror attack made me realize that life was short and could be cut even shorter. Watching the towers collapse put everything into perspective. Life was short, too short for regrets. Too short for loneliness. I had spent so much time building a life, a business, a marriage, only to watch it all unravel. And yet, J still held out his hand, promising we could start again. Maybe it was foolish. Maybe it was hope. But I wanted to believe in second chances.

Suddenly, all the things I thought mattered (work and money) felt small. What was I holding onto? Anger? Fear of the unknown? I had built a life only to watch it unravel, and yet, I wasn't sure how to move forward. What I did know was that I didn't like being alone. I missed taking care of someone, cooking for more than just myself. I didn't get married to get divorced. Plus, living alone wasn't my favorite thing. Maybe we could find a way back to each other. Maybe we could start over.

J suggested I sell our home in Fullerton and give the proceeds to his Dad. Then, Dad would send us the money after we got to Hawaii so we could buy a lot and build something on it.

After I sold the house, Joe, our attorney, recorded it in his Dad's name and gave Dad the money. It's called a constructive trust. Unfortunately for me, nothing was put in writing. Hindsight is twenty-twenty.

For the next three months, I meticulously packed and labeled the contents of our house and sold things that I thought we wouldn't need and wouldn't take with us. One of the things that needed to be sold was his old Mercedes, which had an impressive 500,000 miles on it. It was a classic, still running with its original engine. He liked to tell the story of how Mercedes-Benz had even given him an award for reaching such a high number of original miles—a testament to the car's durability and engineering.

Since J used to pack our trucks for catering, it made sense for him to come back from Hawaii to handle packing the shipping container. We chose Matson, the largest shipping company, and I hoped the best. They dropped off a 24-foot container at the house and were to pick it up once it was packed.

J was a master packer, but after hours and hours of packing, I went outside and saw that the container was full, and the driveway was also full of things that weren't in the container and needed to be. He told me to go back inside, which I did. When I came back out hours later, everything was in the container. I was shocked but relieved that somehow he had made it all fit.

November 8

We moved to the Big Island. When we landed in Hilo, we went from the airport to Big Island Toyota and picked up a white 2001 Echo, stick shift, sight unseen (a first for me) with $15,000 cash. It turned out to be a terrific little car and great for gas economy. Gas on the Big Island was très expensive. And hold its value? Boy, howdy, this car did. I found that out years later when I sold it.

2002

January

They say timing is everything and I'm here to attest to that! We found a lot right on the front of the Seaview subdivision. The best part? No one could ever build in front of us. Amazing. Too good to be true. Ocean view as far as the eye could see. J's dad wired us the money from our house so we could purchase it.

There are two types of lava found on the Big Island: **pahoehoe** and **a'a**. Pahoehoe lava moves and cools slowly, creating a smooth, ropy surface. In contrast, a'a lava, which formed the lot where we lived, moves and cools quickly, leaving behind a rough, jagged surface.

The Big Island is known for rain, but after I moved to Seaview, we experienced a full month of nonstop downpour that everyone said felt extreme, even by Hawaiian standards. I knew that Hilo was considered one of the wettest cities in the US, getting anywhere from 120 to 160 inches of rain annually, but what we got was ridiculous. We spent most of the time hunkered down under the blankets, trying to watch satellite TV, but when it stormed, the feed kept going in and out. We lived in our little Dolphin RV beside the ocean filled with leaping dolphins.

We lived in what I called "tent city," with two 10 x 20 white canopies with sidewalls set up right next to the motorhome. High-end camping, no glamping! J built a kitchen on pallets over the lava. I challenge ANYONE to pack up all their belongings and camp for six months. At first, it's fun, then it's a little frustrating, and then you get used to it and cope. After it's over, you look back and only remember the fun parts because you are grateful for the growth part.

Starting over sounded romantic in theory. In reality, it was exhausting. Everything we owned was crammed into a shipping container, and we were about to build a home from scratch with no real plan, no experience, and barely any money. But standing on our lot, looking out at the endless ocean, I felt something I hadn't in years: possibility. A fresh start. A blank canvas. Maybe, just maybe, we could build something better this time.

We needed to decide what style of house we wanted before we could draw up plans, so we had many discussions, drove around the subdivisions looking at houses, and spoke with many people. We learned about and met an architect, Daniel Bona, who lived in the next subdivision. He and J decided, "A man's home is his … castle." Thus CastleInHawaii (CIH) was born.

When people move to Hawaii and intend to build a house, typically, the first step is purchasing a lot of land. Since building takes time, many people camp on the property while constructing the garage. Then they move into it while they build. This gradual approach allows homeowners to be on-site throughout the process, which is especially helpful given the logistics and costs involved in construction on the Big Island.

After J first convinced me to move, he said he'd "throw up a garage in a couple of weeks." In reality the garage took from January to June, SIX MONTHS. It was so lovely we knew we would never use it as a garage. It was two stories. The last thing to do was paint. During the final week, I told him that if he didn't hurry and finish, I was moving in, painted or not. We named it the Artist's Carriage House, or CH for short. We lived in it as we built the main house and knew instinctively the CH would make a great rental space for families.

We kept building, little by little. When we made money, we bought materials and built. We built the main three-story building year after year. The two ground-floor rooms were suites meant for rental and were the first to be completed. The area in between them was a kitchen for the guests, which we called the breezeway kitchen. Our apartment was on the second and third floors. On the second floor, the front door opened into our living room and our kitchen, with a half bath off to the side. I asked J to build small shelving on one wall in the bathroom so I could display my 20-plus antique snow globes. The third floor was our bedroom and bathroom featuring a jacuzzi tub. The windows in the bathroom were vertical, rainbow-colored windows, inspired by the Mormon church, and overlooked the courtyard. My office and the laundry room were also on the third floor.

February

Hawaii requires a strict four-month quarantine to prevent rabies from entering the state, which we all believed was nonsense and just a money-making scheme. There were no predators, no snakes, and hardly any wildlife—except for the occasional mongoose. Malibu (Bu Kitty) and

Molly (old, long-haired GSD) made it through quarantine but it was difficult for them being in a cage. I visited every day and stayed for hours. Now they are home with us, digging their new digs, cruising and exploring.

The following is my typical schedule:

4:30-5:30 a.m.: Wake up just before the sun. I'm an early bird, so this is a good thing. Have coffee, take a short walk, or do a 10-minute "AB" (abdominal) tape or a 45-minute aerobic tape like "The Firm," my favorite.

6-7 a.m.: I start my workday at my desk, speaking to clients in California. I design parties, plan events, create menus, and coordinate entertainment. I fax, they fax, we all fax.

9 a.m.: When it is noon in California, and my clients are at lunch, I take a break and do some gardening, watering plants, or preparing dinner until people return from lunch.

10-11 a.m.: I am back on the phone until about 2 p.m. when most of my clients since they are on Pacific time finish work and go home, which is 5 p.m. on the West Coast.

2-5 p.m.: More gardening, walking the dog, knitting, reading, making ice cream. The world is my oyster. Mom taught me how to knit, so I feel closer to her when I do. I miss her, even though I call her often.

Every night of the week, there is a different activity (or not). Monday is (what Mormons call) Family Home Evening. We might watch a video or play board games and make and have a special dessert. On Tuesdays, my husband has Boy Scouts. The Mormon church needs people to serve in the Scouts, and it is my husband's pleasure to do so. I get a night to myself! On Wednesdays, a group of us might go to the farmer's market or dinner and a movie. On Thursdays and Fridays, we do whatever or nothing. On Saturdays, there's yoga at 8 a.m. at the Wellness

Retreat, about a mile or so from my house, after which I typically go to the farmer's market in Hilo, a 45-minute drive to shop and do errands. I actually don't care for yoga but enjoy being social. On Sundays, church is from 9 to noon, and then we hit the beach. It's a clothing-optional beach, but it's *not* optional for me—I don't want to scare people off the beach! And then I like to make a special Sunday night dinner, perhaps with the missionaries or an invited guest or two. I love to cook for people!

Last year in California, my schedule was:

I got up between 5 and 6 a.m. and started working at my desk or running like a mad person all day. I would get home between 7 and 11 p.m., depending on if we had an event. Then I dropped into bed and passed out by midnight while watching TV shows I taped on the VCR.

Holidays were a nightmare—since it was my livelihood, I never decorated my house for Christmas or any holiday for that matter and would rather be in bed. I hated to go to parties unless I was being paid to be there.

The point is, you'd think losing every-thing—my business and, for a while, my husband—would be the worst thing that could happen to a person. That's what I thought as I was going through it. In actuality, it was the best thing that ever happened. All I lost was an amazing disposable yearly income. I was a spoiled JAP (Jewish American Princess, a term used back in the day; I'm pretty sure using it today is unacceptable). I had weekly manicures, pedicures, massages, car washes, personal trainer, monthly hair appointments, and drove a Lincoln Navigator. If I saw it and wanted it, I bought it. I was a type A personality that few people could tolerate being around. Now, I am a relaxed, happy, blissful per-son who takes time to listen and learn. Instead of a Navigator, I drive a Toyota

Echo—probably one of the smallest cars made and gets 44 miles to the gallon! I adore it.

I went from hardly ever smiling to always smiling. From trying to run people off the road and get them out of my way to allowing drivers to get ahead of me. From breathing pollution 24/7 to breathing clean, sweet, fragrant, air and blooms from abundant plumeria and tuberose, my favorites. From buying everything I saw to seeing very few things I want or think I want. What you own owns you! I went from a 1,800-square-foot home to an 800-square-foot home. From over 1,700 cellular minutes a month to 200-500. From getting up and putting on makeup and a uniform or business attire to getting up and never putting on makeup and wearing shorts and T-shirts every day, except Sunday when I wear a dress for a couple of hours to go to church. I gave up all shoes except Birks (Birkenstock), Crocs, and sneakers.

Living in Paradise can get a little lonely as most of the people here are eccentric, or they are hermits, and there just aren't that many people here, period! You REALLY have to co-exist with yourself comfortably.

March

On March 17, 2002, our castle made it to the front page of the local newspaper. There was a festival or some sort of event happening in the park across the road from the castle, and the photographer snapped a pic that caught our house in the background.

It seems you can just mention "the castle" and people have either heard of it or seen it. I was in line at the Natural Health food store and heard people talking about it. That was surreal. Helicopter tours hover pretty regularly above our house. I can imagine them saying, "Here's the only castle in the state, right next to the lava flow." Being right next to the flow did make me a little (a lot!) nervous.

At least three times a week, I notice people stopping to take pictures of the house. It always makes me laugh. I start imagining myself wearing a crown and posing for them, just for fun. I wished I had one of those paper crowns from Burger King. We've even joked about building a throne in one of the bathrooms in the main house.

One day in Hilo, I happened upon a group of people and German shepherds doing protection training in a park. I heard a sharp, commanding voice echo across the park, followed by deep, powerful barks. Intrigued, I walked closer and saw a bunch of German shepherds, their eyes locked on a man in a thick padded suit. One in particular was standing about 50 feet from the "helper". He shouted something in German, and in an instant, the dog lunged forward, teeth sinking into the sleeve, holding firm until given the signal to release. It was controlled, precise, powerful. I felt a thrill rush through me. This wasn't just training—it was a partnership, an understanding between dog and handler. Schutzhund is called a triathlon for dogs, combining obedience, protection, and tracking.

The official website describes Schutzhund as a sport that evaluates a dog's intelligence and usefulness. It tests their mental stability, endurance, structure, scenting ability, willingness to work, courage, and trainability. A key component of the training is the "out" command (**aus** in German) when the dog must release the sleeve upon command. Failure to do so can result in the dog being discouraged from breeding.

Molly was getting older, and the thought of losing her weighed on me. I knew I wanted to bring another dog into our lives before she passed, hoping a puppy might help keep her young at heart and give her someone to play with. When I found a breeder with a litter on the way, it felt like the right decision. She gave me first pick, and I chose a boy, named him Samson after my grandfather, Sam. In Jewish tradition, we honor the deceased by passing on their name, or at least the first letter of the name.

December

I paid the breeder $1,100. Unfortunately, Sam really wasn't a qualified Schutzhund prospect, but as a newbie, I had no idea. He was the best I thought I could find on the Big Island. There were breeders on Oahu, but it would have been more money for the dog, plus airfare. I needed to start somewhere.

The best thing was getting to know him from three days old until I got to bring him home at 49 days, which is the recommended time frame. I read every training book I could get my hands on. The monks of New Skete wrote a tremendous one called *The Art of Training Your Dog*. There was also a wealth of books and DVDs on Schutzhund, and I bought a bunch.

2003

In my community of Seaview, nicknames and aliases were the norm. Women had names like Rainbow, Aloha, Geranium, and Spirit. For as long as I can remember, I've wanted a different name, though I could never quite pinpoint why. If naming my animals was difficult, naming myself was nearly impossible.

When I went to Camp Wishe, I gave myself the nickname Scamp. Well, it was accurate, but really? Scamp? I guess I owned it from an early age. Just call me Bliss from now on, and we'll see how it goes. To me, bliss meant living an authentic life—choosing joy over obligation, passion over resentment. I was finally doing what I wanted, not what I thought I should be doing. I was living my dream and, in the process, relearning how to live.

Bliss felt like euphoria—colors more vivid, the ocean air sweeter, sunsets more breathtaking than I ever imagined. But paradise came with a price. The bugs? Enormous. The roaches? They flew, which was unnerving!

Living in Paradise had its tradeoffs. I likened it to living on the frontier, the Wild West, or the outback. The nearest gas station or store to buy milk was 15 minutes away. The closest (competent) doctor, vet, or paramedic? Who knew, and I hoped never to have to find out.

The best thing was planting a pineapple top in the lava, and a year later, you had a pineapple to eat. When we got the property, I immediately bought a mango tree. When it bore fruit a few years later, we had a little ceremony, sitting under the tree, cutting and eating the mango.

There was no county water in my community, just catchment. When I first arrived, I thought it was cool that everyone had above-ground pools. As it turns out, those "pools" were actually water catchment tanks.

There were inconveniences, like no DSL or cable modem, but that was the tradeoff. It was paradise, after all. And there weren't enough people on the island, maybe 150,000, for anyone to care. Not enough business for them. It took longer to email and to download, but so what?

One of the best things about living here was never seeing a police car or speed trap. The cops all drove their own cars with a blue light on top. They were mostly Hawaiians, but I had seen one haole (pronounced howlie). They called white people haole. If you weren't insane, you never had to deal with the cops. You mostly saw them at construction sites where they redid the roads, wearing white gloves and orange vests. Only one road went all around the island, so it was hard to get lost.

I couldn't explain how it felt to once again be in an actual waterproof structure—our home, our castle. Having lived with virtually nothing for the past six months, it seemed that even after selling most of my stuff, I STILL had way too much crap! A lot of the things I was unpacking had to be repacked until we moved out of the garage and into the main house, if that ever happened. We were just $100,000 short. And if it never happened, that was ok too. I didn't want to move an inch, go to town, or shop, even though I needed to. I hadn't picked up my mail in days. We had a box in Pahoa, but who cared? Who needed mail anyway? Usually, it was mostly bills. Not like when we wrote letters back in the day.

One of the wonderful things about food in Hawaii, aside from the ability to plant and grow your own, was that much of what you bought was locally grown, freshly picked, and organic. Papaya, my favorite fruit, became a daily staple;

I even propagated the seeds to grow our own papaya trees. Though food costs were higher, the payoff in health was well worth it. My cholesterol levels dropped dramatically—from over 300 to 198, within the recommended range of 200 or below.

For breakfast, we ate fruit, yogurt, or cottage cheese. Lunch was a sandwich or a salad. Dinner was a huge salad, some protein (beef, fish, or chicken), and some starch (rice, pasta, or potatoes), with way smaller portions than we used to eat. And lots of garlic! Roasted, grated, in and on everything. Lots of freshly brewed green and other herbal teas. I had never felt so healthy or powerful in my life. I thought I had eaten well before, but now I knew I did!

The style of this house/castle was probably the most difficult and expensive we could have picked. Of course, it was. The outside coating was quite a process. First, J screwed foam blocks on the wood walls, then he slapped on mud, and finally, he sprayed it with a plastic that looked like stone. I was documenting everything with pictures and video. Permits, red tape, and plans galore! Plus, the TIME it took! Expensive? Boy howdy. But building your own home? Priceless!

Seeing nothing but a peaceful ocean all around and smelling the fragrant ocean air, how could one not feel happy and at peace? My dog Molly was at my feet, with me constantly, instead of being the "yard" dog she used to be. She was right behind me if I went toward the car, knowing she was going for a ride!

Our cat Punkin curled up in various places at various times, waiting for a kiss and a pat as I went by. The cats in California—Malibu, Samantha, and Tiffany—might have been left alone for days while we worked. The animals I loved had been neglected as I spun my wheels, getting nowhere fast, back on the mainland. If you ever call it the States, you would have gotten your head handed to you. Hawaii IS part of the states.

The hardest tradeoff was missing my mama, dear friends, and the ferrets, which I had to re-home. Other than that, my soul soared. I hoped everyone would come visit me before they and I died!

Aloha, Bliss (Sheri)

2006

December 31

I took Sam for a walk around the community, but something was off. He was lagging behind me, which was unlike him. People were setting off fireworks, but he was used to training with gunshots, so I knew the sound of the fireworks wasn't what was disturbing him. A knot formed in my stomach, sensing something wasn't right. We returned home, and despite my unease, we went to bed. I hoped the feeling would pass by morning.

2007

January 1

When I woke up, I went downstairs, and Sam looked at me like, "Mama, help!" For some reason, I looked at his tummy and saw it was distended. I immediately called the vet, who told me to bring him right in.

Speeding up the hill toward Hilo, a bird slammed into my windshield. I can only assume it died, but I wasn't about to stop the ambulance run I was on. Can you spell foreshadowing?

An x-ray revealed his spleen was five times its normal size, so it had to be removed immediately. The doctor told me, "You can probably take him home tomorrow." Was he delusional, thinking I would leave my boy there alone? He headed back to perform the surgery on Sam, while I paced anxiously in the waiting room.

An hour later, my world collapsed. The vet came out, his face telling me what I didn't want to hear. Sam died of a heart attack in post-op. He's dead? It can't be. I had to see him. The sobs that escaped my throat were surreal. They couldn't be coming from me. I couldn't control them. They just kept coming, raw and unstoppable. After a time of sitting there wailing and feeling helpless, I realized I didn't want to keep the vet and his assistant away from their families any longer on New Year's Day, but I just couldn't breathe, move or compose myself. The grief swallowed me whole.

In the end, it was a thousand-dollar surgery for a dead dog. I paid the bill and we loaded his hundred-pound body onto a stretcher and into the back of my car where, just a day ago, his head hung out with his tongue waving in the wind, ridiculously cute.

The drive home was endless, and the silence deafening. I was numb in disbelief. My boy was in the back of my car, DEAD. When we pulled into the driveway of the house, Molly greeted the car, and for a minute, I panicked. Do I let her near so she can smell him, smell death? My gut said yes, so I did.

J walked up to the car when I arrived, and I told him he had to dig a grave. He said little about Sam's death. It took two hours to dig through the lava rock. He dug the grave right next to Malibu, my Bu-Kitty, who knew enough to leave after twenty good, long, fat, and happy years. My other two cats before him, Samantha and Tiffany, also stayed until at least twenty, I think because they didn't want to leave their mama. We'd designated an area in the backyard for a small cemetery. Having a resting place for them here brought some comfort—it was where they belonged, close to me.

After calling the breeder and a few close friends to share the news of Sam's death, I finally lay down around 9 p.m. Somehow, I managed to doze off, but two hours later, I woke up in tears, realizing I had been crying even in my sleep. The disbelief hit me all over again. Twenty-five days later, little had changed. The only difference was I could almost go a whole day without crying. When it was time to try to sleep, the tears poured from both my eyes and my heart. The grief was overwhelming, likely because I had known him since he was just a few days old. Losing him felt unbearably hard. He had been by my side every moment, 24/7.

The days were empty, and the nights were unbearable without him. The depression was so oppressive I could barely muster enough strength to speak above a whisper. What happened to my life? Sam was dead. This was not supposed to happen! Not this way. Parents are supposed to die first. He was taken in the prime of his life, leaving so much untold potential. I felt like I'd been run over by a truck, just regained consciousness, and the morphine drip was doing nothing to dull the pain. I felt like an amputee. My arm was missing, and no one noticed.

A month later, when the tears finally slowed—because they never really stop—I reached out to a Schutzhund judge. She knew a dog for me in Germany.

I asked her how much. After she told me and I got off the floor and paid, she "made it so" (Star Trek's Captain Picard's favorite term). I spent my life savings that I had hidden under my mattress and kept secret even from my husband.

February 14

Let the spending begin! To say the least, the sport of Schutzhund was expensive. Plus I had a lot to learn. His German name was Relax vom Struwwelpeter. Relax was pronounced "Raylocks," so I decided his call name would be Ray. I also decided he should have the Hawaiian name Rayla.

Since quarantine was four months, I arranged for Ray to be flown from Germany to Cali to spend three months continuing his training with Max, the judge's husband in Denver. Then he could go to quarantine for the last month on the Big Island so we could bond.

Ray flew into LAX, and I flew in from Hawaii to meet him. He arrived on Valentine's Day, a date I'll never forget because it's when we fell in love. We spent the weekend at a motel before flying to Denver. Since Ray didn't "speak" English and I didn't know German, I spent that weekend honeymoon researching German commands online and teaching him their English translations.

In Germany, it's common practice for many dog owners and breeders to feed dogs raw chicken, which was what Ray was used to. When he went to Max, who trained up to twenty dogs at a time, I didn't feel comfortable asking Max to go buy chicken for Ray. I allowed him to feed kibble during those three months. Looking back, I can't help but attribute some of Ray's later health issues to that decision (cue the Jewish guilt).

Ray was 21 months old when he got out of quarantine and got to me on the Big Island. The county ran a kennel facility in Keaau specifically for that purpose, and it was about twenty minutes from the castle. The last month he was in quarantine, I spent four to six hours a day with him, building rapport.

I made a flyer to let people know Ray was available for stud services. The minute he got out of jail, uh, I mean quarantine, he had three dates to stand at stud.

June 16

It became apparent that the Echo wouldn't work for training. Big German shepherd in a tiny car, no bueno. Also, the dogs are supposed to be brought to training in a kennel (crate) in the car and kept in the kennel during training. They learn by watching. I bought him a Toyota Rav4, and the first thing I bought for the Rav was a people mover (the metal grate that goes around the front bumper and headlights). I like a tough-looking car, especially after the Echo.

And while I didn't actually name her, I did refer to her as a her, kind of like a boat.

While I was building rapport with my new son, J was building a spec house just up the road at the top of the subdivision. A "spec" house (short for speculative) is a house that is built by a builder with the hope that it will sell once it is completed. The house is not built for a specific buyer, but rather constructed with general market appeal, and is put up for sale after construction. J called it the Sweetheart Cottage (SC). It took him about a year to finish, and it was adorable even though it was built in a puka (Hawaiian word for hole).

When Ray got out of quarantine, I tried to feed him raw, but it was difficult for me. I put him on raw in the morning and a mix of kibble and homemade organic stew with cooked meat and veggies in the evening. That was no better according to Dr. J, who was my vet for over thirty years in SoCal. He wrote a book on nutrition and feeding raw. He immortalized Ray on the cover, for which I will always be grateful. PaleoPet.guide.

2008

The economy tanked everywhere, taking our plans down with it. We had finished building the SC, after investing about $200,000—plus countless hours of sweat equity. Once completed, we planned to list it, and we would finally be flush! The collapse of the economy, the recession, or whatever you call it, made that impossible.

Desperate for a solution, I had a "brilliant" idea to run an essay contest to win the home so we could recoup our investment. Gambling was not permitted in Hawaii so we hired an attorney to fact-check to make sure it would be copacetic. I created a website: WinHawaiianHome.com. I got a piece on a local news station and posted it on my YouTube channel. I acquired my own personal troll. He had all the time in the world to diminish the contest and talk smack about us. That's what happens when you put yourself out there, I guess.

I resisted at first, but eventually, I finally "came around" and realized that raw was the only way to feed. When Ray came to me on the Big Island in July 2007, his coat was glossy, full, and thick. But within a year, everything changed. Bloody hot spots. Flaky skin. Scabs. His elbows were rough and cracked like elephant skin. Every part of his body was affected, so I eliminated wheat, kibble, all grains, and everything Dr. J recommended. I tried shampoos and products from allergicpet.com and spent over $1,500 during the first year on remedies. I kept track with pictures of each new symptom and flare-up. Then one day, his left paw went lame.

I put him on bed rest; a week later, the problem was pretty much gone and he was able to walk without a limp. I did a HESKA test on him for allergens, hoping it would let me know what he was allergic to, if anything, so I could resolve his skin issues. Ragweed and dust mites came back positive. Things I couldn't exactly eliminate. This was a freaking nightmare.

2009

I built a website for the castle, and by late 2009, **CastleInHawaii.com** was officially open for guests. Bookings trickled in for the two lower-level suites while we scrambled to finish our apartment upstairs.

Our first guest was an influencer, likely one of the first ever, who helped promote our vacation rental. The horrible part was that we didn't have curtains on the suite windows yet. **What. Were. We. Thinking?**

I envisioned and designed purple velvet curtains, which gave a regal touch, and my girlfriend, a seamstress, brought my vision to life. Unfortunately, it was too late for our first guest.

My husband's bipolar symptoms resurfaced again—major déjà vu. But I still didn't have a name for it. It left me feeling helpless and overwhelmed. I begged him to get help, to get diagnosed, pouring all my hope into the possibility of finding a solution. His steadfast refusal felt like a personal rejection, deepening my despair and leaving me grappling with a profound sense of isolation. The man I married was slipping away, and I was powerless to stop it. And left me more alone than ever.

The 2010s

September 6

I sent this letter to Mary, Ray's breeder in Germany. I even translated it into German:

> I'm writing with a broken heart, not out of malice, but because I thought you should know what's happening with Relax. I don't expect you to do anything. It just is what it is.

I wanted a Schutzhund dog. What I have is a dog who was once athletic and strong but now struggles to climb stairs. My bedroom is on the second floor, but soon, we'll be moving to the third. He won't be able to follow me without pain.

My last dog died of torsion at just four years old, in his prime. Later, I learned that every pup from his litter had died of one issue or another. Now I wonder— would you allow me to contact Relax's littermates? Are they even still alive?

In August 2007, he started having horrible skin problems and hot spots. I have pictures of his whole back that was bloody. I finally found out he has a low thyroid and needs a pill twice a day, which could be contributing to or causing the skin problem. I had to put him on steroids for almost a year, which was HORRIBLE, and finally got him off of them by switching to a drug that costs $6 a pill. But more importantly, it prevented us from doing Schutzhund because I couldn't put a pinch collar on him due to his raw and sensitive neck.

Then we went swimming, and the next day, he was in such great pain that I took him to the vet. I wanted to rule out torsion. He did not have torsion, but they thought he had a blockage. It happened again right before we were scheduled to go to California, so I took him to Dr. J, my vet of twenty years, and he diagnosed an enlarged spleen.

After looking at his x-rays, Dr. J told me his spine was narrowing around the cord and pressing on nerves, causing the pain. It is called stenosis, which is something like sciatica in humans. Spinal stenosis may affect the cervical, thoracic, or lumbar spine. In some cases, it may be present in all three places in the same patient. Lumbar spinal stenosis results in low back pain and pain or abnormal sensations in the legs, thighs, and feet or loss of bladder and bowel control.

Dr. J sent me to a specialist vet, who was used by a Schutzhund judge. He did the ultrasound and told me he could fix it for $4,000-6,000. He needed an MRI and surgery. Even if I had that kind of money lying around, is this something I want to put this boy through? Right now, we live day to day. I'm reluctant to let him exert himself because I don't want to cause him pain. I haven't even been walking him every morning, which totally SUCKS. This dog is brilliant, and we have developed a very close connection. At times, I think he can read my mind. He is neutral to everything except ME. He never takes his eyes off me. He loves our three cats and our mini dachshund. He is the PERFECT service dog. I am heartbroken. That's my story. I was wondering if you would write back and tell me your thoughts.

Of course, she never replied.

* * *

THE MARRIAGE REF IS NOW CASTING

Jerry Seinfeld, NBC, and the producers of Super Nanny now bring you ... *The Marriage Ref*: A reality series where couples and a relationship referee help squabbling couples make peace. Created by Seinfeld himself, this is relationship advice ... with a comic twist.

The Marriage Ref is searching the country for outgoing and opinionated couples in long-term relationships who are willing to appear on national television and have a long-standing argument or issue that must be resolved. No problem is too small!

Is there an object, a person, or a habit (e.g., a computer, a pet, a friend, the remote control) that is a third wheel in your relationship and causes a problem? Does your partner have an annoying, obnoxious habit or item that causes fights? Does your partner do things like withhold sex after a fight? Whatever you argue about, we want to hear from you. Tell us why you absolutely need a Marriage Ref to weigh in and decide who is RIGHT and who is WRONG.

It sounded intriguing, so I applied. Here's what I sent:

> J and Sheri have been married for twenty years. They don't need a referee for one fight. They need a live-in ref. Full-time.

> They live on the Big Island of Hawaii at the CastleInHawaii, a home J built for his queen. Their court includes Merlin (his white cat), Gwenivere (her black cat), Ray (her well-trained German shepherd), and Bruiser (his mini-weenie, a stubborn and selectively deaf mini Doxie).

> The king and queen couldn't be more different. They agree on one thing. They don't agree on anything. Now they are arguing over WHICH argument the Marriage Ref should decide on!

1. He's Mormon. She's Jewish. Kinda like Larry King and his wife, except he's Jewish, and she's Mormon. Aren't they getting a divorce now?

2. THE DOGS: The king has Bruiser, a sausage. The queen has Ray, a well-trained German shepherd who listens and obeys. The weenie is exactly like the king and doesn't even listen to him! And the king doesn't listen to the queen. She wants him to train his dog, and he thinks it's cute that the dog doesn't listen and "has a mind of his own."

3. THE DOGS/ANIMALS, PART 2: The queen believes the best nutrition for the canines is raw food (chicken, sheep, beef, ahi, pork), so that's what she feeds them. It is arduous, messy, and time-consuming. The king refuses to feed the dogs, even his own dog.

4. THE DOGS/ANIMALS, PART 3: FOOD WARS. Ray wants Bruiser's food, the cats want Ray's food, and Bruiser turns up his nose at ALL food. He is super picky UNLESS (drum roll, please) there is green tripe mixed in. Have you ever SMELLED green tripe? Actually, the only food Bruiser will accept is the king's. The king feeds his dog from the table, which is UNACCEPTABLE to the queen.

5. FOOD FIGHT: The king eats junk food; the queen avoids it like the plague. She takes supplements, but he would never touch supplements. He's a meat and potatoes man, and she'd be a vegetarian if she weren't married to him. She makes smoothies and healthy breakfasts. He eats donuts for breakfast, and the fur flies.

6. FOOD & NUTRITION, PART 2: And why should the queen always cook and feed EVERYBODY? This

man used to be the chef of their catering company and cooked for and fed thousands of people. Now she can't even get him to cook ONE meal for his wife.

7. They're both Pisces. The only thing they have in common. And if astrology is right, two Pisces should NEVER be married.

8. I guess if the royals had to pick one issue, it's that the queen is always doing stuff around the castle. When she asks the king for help, what's his answer? "NO!" or "When I feel like it." He's the king, and he's on vacation (floating in the moat, watching the whales go by, etc.)

Why are we the "perfect" couple for your show? Since we live in paradise, that's a great tax-deductible way for producers to recharge and vacation without admitting it! There are two suites in the castle, and we will provide them to the producers at no charge during their stay. PS: The queen will be in Southern California from June 18 if you would like an audience with us. The king stays home, so let him eat cake. He lives on Planet J.

We didn't make the cut. Probably for the best.

2011

I connected with a woman, Lin, who was in Waipio. She was from Chicago and was having a #MeToo, although we didn't call it that then, the term had yet to be "invented." She needed to escape and be safe. I invited her to stay at the castle. She stayed for three and a half months. Lin wrote a post on her blog:

> Subject: Picture perfect view @ CastleinHawaii

Aloha! I have been enjoying my stay at the gorgeous castle by the sea! The ocean is much closer than I expected. I can hear the calming waves as I go to sleep. It is significantly more relaxed than the pounding swells in Waipio! A moat doubles as a lap pool with a water treadmill, a hot tub on the pool deck, and my personal peaceful, picture-perfect lanai.

February 11

A tsunami hit the Big Island while I was on the mainland. I had a "sitter" at the castle, but he was useless. I knew that unless you lived on the island or were connected with your neighbors, you wouldn't know what to do to batten down the hatches. I got there the day after a hurricane came through and was able to put the place back together. Things had blown around; the pool was filthy, but it was just minor stuff.

October 17

I started a journal called *What Can I Do but Write* because, at that point, writing felt like my only option. My secret therapy. I was going to call it "Miserable in Paradise," but that was horrible since I always tried to be grateful. Wasn't that the opposite of miserable?

I was unhappily married, as I'm sure millions of people are. I felt like I was alone. This was not what I signed up for. So rather than throwing myself off the cliff in front of my house, I thought I'd try writing.

MY JOURNAL

Welcome to my journal. This is my personal therapy. NO ONE is welcome. **Kapu** (Hawaiian for keep out!)

Writing this journal became my therapy. Putting everything into words helped me make sense of how it all unraveled over the years—one chaotic incident after another, with J and with the islanders. I was just trying to survive, to stay committed to my marriage. But the more things spiraled out of control, the more reactive I became. I felt overwhelmed—by my marriage, by not fully understanding what was really happening with J, by the fallout of J's behavior with the neighbors, and by the daily struggles of island life itself.

I wrote to cope. It was all madness. And yet, there comes a point where things have to change. But as you'll see, the chaos had to fully play out before I could even think about what came next.

I'm 57 years old. All I want is to be joyful, happy, and peaceful. I lived with a husband who acted like he was two years old. Some part of me hated to "bitch," but I could bitch on this private blog. Maybe this would help with my (deepening) depression.

We had been married since 1990. You would have thought we would have learned something by now on how to "just get along" (a term coined by Rodney King in 1992 during the LA riots.) Everything was a struggle, a competition. I thought of him as living on Planet J while I lived on Planet Earth. I know I am not perfect; I have flaws, but at least I acknowledged them and tried to do better.

Every day, he'd say things like, "I don't like you" or "You're too critical," and then he'd turn around and criticize me. I wanted someone who uplifted and inspired me, not someone who dragged me down. Was that too much to ask? This man cursed at me, called me names, threw things, and broke things. I took pictures and tried to record the incidents, but so what? I lived in constant fear. He never actually hit me. That didn't mean it wasn't abuse.

October 19

Our castle is the most unique place in the state. We've been in Hawaii for ten years and have been working on it all that time. If we'd had the cash, it would've been done long ago. J was an artist, but everything cost three times what it should have.

We prayed for enough capital to "finish" it. A couple contacted us. Ruth and Leo wanted to move from the East Coast and get away from the horrible winters for an extended period. I didn't think they would be able to live in a suite for an extended period of time since it was just one room, a bathroom, and a patio, so I said no. It was too small. I turned them away and then thought, *Are you CRAZY? This is what you were PRAYING for—a long-term renter.* They could stay in the Carriage House if we could finish it by the time they wanted to arrive.

I called her back after a few days, and she had already found another place. After an hour or so of conversation, long, boring story short, she decided to come and stay since they didn't give any money for the other place. They made it possible for us to FINALLY finish by paying four months' rent in advance.

Someone once said, "Sometimes, God wants to give you something new, but your hands are too full to receive it." Though it can be painful to let go, He's trying to place something even better in your hand—if only you'd release what's already there. People who need a divorce go through that same struggle. You will get over it, but you just can't imagine how. After twenty years, I was struggling with that concept. I never should have married J, but I couldn't imagine how to change that without more chaos. We had no marriage; we had a roommate arrangement where I was the maid, assistant, and secretary, and he was the boss. His favorite phrase was: "Listen to me. Do what I tell you." Really?

He called from Hilo and was trying to coerce me to help him make a Haunted Castle. It was only a couple of weeks until Halloween. My idea would be to have enough time to actually plan and do it the following year. I offered that, but he rejected it. I'm too smart to stray from my focus right now. I knew two weeks was not enough time to promote this idea to be successful. I wanted to focus on the remodel, booking jobs with my catering business, or helping him get construction jobs.

Then, he wanted to be Santa at the mall. Seven days a week, for six weeks, ten hours a day, with no "understudy". Really? He told me he didn't care about what I needed or wanted, but I should make HIS needs and wants MY priority.

October 20

J left before 6 a.m., and now it was almost 1 p.m. Seven whole hours of quiet and peace. So, the maid had been cleaning (detailing) the kitchen. And by maid, I mean me. And writing. The only thing about him not being here was the wasted time for our deadline to finish the CH before Ruth and Leo arrived. He is doing haunted castle stuff instead of focusing on his commitment getting the space ready for them.

October 21

Today, I got out of bed at 5:30 a.m., and J announced he would be leaving for Hilo in 15 minutes. I went to the kitchen to make a cooler of food so he didn't have to buy anything. I made him a healthy breakfast of nuts, made sure he had bottles of water, etc., and lunch meat or a hard-boiled egg. He said he'd only be gone for a "couple of hours." Yeah, right, I've heard that before. He came into the kitchen and announced, "I'm leaving now." I said, "Your egg is almost ready." Usually, he'll just leave after I've done all the work and leave the cooler (sweet guy). Then, if that happens, he'll let me run after him, begging him to take it so as not to waste money, my time, or the food. Well, this time, he actually waited the one minute for me to finish cooling and peeling the egg, and he took the cooler. Wasn't I lucky?

Yesterday, I asked him to get a gallon of milk since he drinks 90 percent of it, and he called whining that he didn't have enough cash to get it. When he got home, I looked in his "murse" (man purse), which was what we called his fanny pack, and there was $5. Well, ok, in Hawaii, it won't buy a gallon, but it would get a quart …? Before you get the wrong idea that I was a snoop, which I probably was anyway out of necessity, these past ten years, when I asked for his receipts, he always said: "Get them from my wallet."

Another important thing to me was keeping the stuff we owned safe and having it last as long as possible since we didn't have money to replace things. A case in point is our (2001) Toyota Echo. I protected the seats all those years with seat covers for the front and blankets for the hatchback. The back seats were always down so there was room for Ray and whatever stuff we had to put in it. That way, the seats stayed pristine.

Yesterday, when I went to get into the Echo, the seats were up. There was a stain on the back seat, so I guess he picked up hitchhikers since there was NO other reason for him to lift the seats. And guess who had to scrub out the stain? Three guesses. First two don't count.

When we first started building, there was a gaping hole in the pool deck where the dungeon was going to be. I asked J to put barriers around it so no one would get hurt, especially me. One evening, I went out there and fell ten feet into the dungeon, landing on the concrete below. I compressed my spine so badly that I couldn't move for hours.

Turns out, I had fractured my back. I asked and got an RX (prescription) from my doctor for a service dog, and that was how Ray became my service animal so he could help me get up and steady me.

My opinion is that this man was so damaged by his umpteen stepfathers growing up that this was all he knew. Chaos and battling are normal for him, so he stirred the pot to ensure he had it.

He went to garage sales and bought other people's old, discarded crap and strewed it all around our space. He never asked if I liked it or wanted it. He just dumped it around our home. I hate clutter—glass, vases, nick-nacks, and hideous crap that was probably not worth a nickel, if that. I've had antiques for over 30 years, so this stuff was not acceptable.

This situation caused my stomach to be in knots. I'm usually 135-140 pounds. (Did I really just admit that?) I went down to 128, but it was not the way I would have liked to do it. Don't get me wrong, I love my body temple and always try to honor it despite my foibles and self-medicating, which is ironic.

He stood on his platform and preached about karma and accused me of being negative using small things—like accidentally getting my iPhone wet, which cost us $250 to replace—as examples. Then *he* destroyed Johnny, his 1989 work truck, for no good reason. Here's how it went: I had asked him for weeks to check the oil. One day, I woke up and told him again to check the oil! My gut was telling me something. He never maintained our vehicles anyway, so typically, I was the one that had to. He was going to Hilo that day, and I told him again to check the oil. Thirty-five minutes later, he called me from Hilo and told me the engine blew up. We had replaced the engine from normal wear not even a year ago, costing us $3,000.

On planet J, there was no planning for the future; you just spent whether you had the money or not or borrowed or convinced other people to pay for things. His Karma was backing into other people's cars. That cost us. I asked him to roll his window down when backing up, at the very least, with trailers and/or trucks. Did he consider that? No. Now he had an iPhone, so on top of that, he listened to music with earplugs so he really couldn't hear anything, especially me. Can you spell passive-aggressive?

I decided that "detailing" my kitchen was the prescription to get Zen, so I did. It sparkled. It made me happy. If he walked in there, it would be a mess in two seconds. And if I didn't cook for him, he would go out and spend money to eat. It must be nice. I scrimped and saved and made food to save money. He ate out and spent money that we didn't have. Ok, enough bitching for now. Back to work. No extra charge for the show.

October 22

He asked me, "Where's my allowance?" The man hadn't worked in two months, expected me to pay bills AND give him money to ... go out to eat? Hmmm.

The BS started last night. He slept on the couch. Then in the morning, it started again before I had a chance to grab a freaking cup of coffee. It was about our credit card debt. Yep, we had a ton, but it was not enough to suit him. He called from WallyWorld (what we called Walmart) and started bitching that he didn't have enough credit to buy more crap for the Haunted Castle.

When I got to my desk, I saw he had left work for the secretary (me). He wanted me to type a letter of apology he had handwritten to his ex—ten years ago. A Post-it was attached, saying he needed it typed so he could send it to his daughter. At the very bottom, like an after-thought, he even managed to include a "please."

We owed everyone and their mother. He used his fuzzy logic to get thousands of dollars worth of granite from some poor guy in Pahoa. After he had the granite in his possession, the guy settled on a price of $1,000 for all of it; did he have a choice? It was worth way more. J already had the granite and told me they had a deal.

Before I got to Hawaii, J had catered a wedding for a couple in our ward. There was some kind of misunderstanding. All I knew and found out was that they were angry. He was unclear with everyone he dealt with.

Another example? He did a remodel job for a woman in our ward who now hates him because he ran up $6,000 on her Home Depot card getting materials for our place. I begged him to make a "contract" for her to sign like we always did for a catering job. She took him to court, and she won.

A couple in a nearby subdivision were his next victims. He built a house for them and made such confusing side deals that I had no clue what happened. I'm sure we owed them, but there was no exact figure, and luckily, they didn't come after us.

Everyone "couldn't stand" me because I wanted to be clear. I was a bitch, yet he wore a halo. Fuzzy logic. I love that term. I live with it. At least he was vaguely aware of his issue of being unclear. When I tried to point things out as they were happening, he claimed short-term memory loss. If I tried to give or show him "tools" to help remember things, he didn't want to hear it. For example, if I needed to remember to take something with me, I left it by the door. Right where I would trip over it and thus remember to take it. He walked around it and yelled at me: "Why is this in the way?" I didn't even want to think about all the lost hours I'd spent looking for things he took, borrowed, or used and either left where he used it or didn't put it back.

He accused me of criticizing him and was doing the exact same thing to me ten minutes later. He said that we stayed together because he loved me. I was sure that's not how you show love—yelling and cursing and name-calling. Our neighbor, a good friend, asked me, "Why is J doing the haunted castle when he has so much to do to make the deadline for the tenants who are coming?" I laughed. I couldn't respond but my brain shouted: EGO. He took all the air out of the room or the neighborhood if he was outside. He stood up in church to give his testimony. It was a Morman thing. He said he was Einstein reincarnated or something to that effect. Afterward, a girlfriend asked me, "What the heck was that?"

We studied Kabbalah, which taught us that you are supposed to abolish ego. He went to church to try to learn how to be like Jesus. He could have fooled me. He spoke to me in front of whoever happened to be around like I was an insect. I couldn't say he treated me like a dog because his favorite saying was, "I wish my wife would treat me like she treats her dog." He said, "Don't touch MY stuff," and then ten minutes later, it was OUR stuff if that fit the situation. His favorite saying when we were in California was "delayed gratification." Words to live by? Not anymore.

October 28

Shaka: That unmistakable pinky and thumb salute was the ultimate symbol of aloha and local culture in Hawaii. Interpreted to mean "hang loose" or "right on." The shaka was a constant reminder that it was not the norm to worry or rush in Hawaii. It represented the embodiment of "island style" and signaled that everything was all right. It was like a fist bump or air kiss. Howzit? Wassup? Writing for therapy has helped. I didn't like who I had become, living with J. I didn't want to stoop to his level, and often, that was just what I found myself doing. It sucked. I saw him trip on something recently; I pretended I didn't see it. One day, he said jokingly: "You probably spit in my food." Darlin', the way you acted, you should be glad I didn't poison your food!

He commanded: "Manifest cash." Then, when I did? Case in point: there was a lovely couple here from California. They had booked in May before we knew we were going to have to remodel. He got up in the middle of the night to work and made a racket using power tools. OMG.

I begged and pleaded, "DON'T WAKE UP THE GUESTS." His comment? "You shouldn't have booked them when I needed to do construction." They DID book, they WERE here, and we needed to keep our commitment for them to have a great and memorable stay. Well, it would be memorable, all right, but for the wrong reasons.

We contracted and promised a view of the ocean from their lanai. Then came J's obsession with the Haunted Castle. He put three huge banners on the fence that obliterated the gorgeous ocean view. When I mentioned that they were not going to be happy, his comment was, "They won't mind." Really? Was that what he thought? The girl was beyond angry, and thankfully, she took pity on me when she saw what I was going through. She didn't pack her bags, demand her money back and run. I bought them a bottle of wine and promised some free nights if they would return, although I thought that was highly unlikely.

He was a BS artist besides being an artist. When he screwed up our books running his construction company with his dad in 2007, the finance and late charges took most of his profit. He would buy or pay for something since the money was coming. Then, when it didn't arrive in time—bouncy bounce, cha-ching. He had wanted to take all our bill-paying money to finance his Haunted Castle. Over my dead body. I had become a mama grizzly, but instead of a cub, it was my survival I was trying to protect. Don't screw with me, dude. I wasn't going down the BK road with him again. I was trying to separate his credit from mine. He hadn't worked in months. And when he did, instead of doing the work himself, he hired his buddy of the moment to do it and make the money and the profit.

He had bought a high cube truck for $2,500 from a church member. It had been sitting ever since he bought it. I don't think he ever used it. Now, it was a glorified tool shed, although it was mostly empty since a majority of the tools were at the SC.

He bought a piece of crap minivan for $1,000. Then he went to an auction and bought a 15-passenger cargo van before we discussed it or sold the old van so we would have the cash to pay for it. He made me put it on my card. Thankfully, I finally sold the old van.

The issue with the club van was that it was a gas guzzler. It was against everything I stood for—not wasting gas or resources, etc. I was trying to "walk the walk" and save the planet. The bad thing about having the van was that it enabled him to go to auctions and buy crap. All the fantastic bargains he had scored on sale on our credit card were now costing more with an added finance charge.

Dear God, didn't you hear my prayers for sanity? He bought a $5 mattress at an auction that they should have paid HIM to cart to the dump. It stank from mold and mildew, and who knows what bugs lurked in that thing. This was what he wanted to put in the remodel for guests?

The Echo needed service, and in addition my Rav's lighter didn't work, which was horrible because I couldn't charge my phone. I went to Goodwill for clothes if I ever wanted or needed something. New low. And it WAS my fault—I couldn't seem to use bleach without getting it all over my clothes.

My needs never got met. So why was I still here? Case in point: all I ever wanted and wished for was a blessing for our property. I set a date of 11/12/11 and sent out a "save the date" email. Now, I had to cancel because of his HC. I was unwilling to do both. The whole community was dead set against the HC.

More waste: I had AT&T as my cell provider, and he went out and bought a Verizon droid … that cost us over $500. He never bothered to learn how to use the phone for a whole year. I didn't know how to work it either since I had an Iphone. I finally got him an iPhone so I could teach him how to use it. Plus, his ringing phone was so important to answer that someone came up behind him in Wally World and stole his wallet. It had cash in it and a $200 gift card for Lowes. Avoiding waste is the biggest thing to me, and he was a waste master.

Why was I still there? I needed to be elsewhere. Death was not the only option or the best option, but I understood why it was so seductive. Some vodka and pills and Aloha Grim Reaper. But if you failed, then you were nuts and into the psych ward you went. They were coming to take me away, haha, hoho, hehe, to the funny farm where life is beautiful all the time.

"Why don't you leave?" If I heard that question one more time from well-meaning loved ones and friends, I was going to pull out all my hair and scream at the top of my lungs—in private, of course, which is what I did by the cliff across the street. At the cliff, I could scream. No one would hear me over the ocean. The waves swallowed my screams. Ray was with me and I wondered what he thought. I knew by his eyes he was worried for his poor mama.

Why didn't I leave? I would have lost what I had worked for these past twenty years. In my own twisted way, was I waiting for one of us to die for the other to be happy?

J had created a work of art. A mirror to put over the sink of the bathroom in the CH. He was too busy to put it up, so I decided I would do it. It was raining, and the walkway was slick. Why, in God's name, did I have to do it then? But I did, and I fell. I was terrified of breaking the mirror. Then he would really have had a reason to blame me for something. I saved it from hitting the floor and shattering at the cost of a gash on my right hand, a tweaked knee, and hitting my head on the doorframe. I was bloody and had a black eye. He pretended to care, but only because he had an audience—his workers. He rushed over, acted concerned, and asked if I was okay. I stared at him in disbelief. "Get away from me," I said, my voice cold. I turned to one of his workers and asked for help getting up, leaving him and the broken mirror behind as I crawled to the couch to lick my wounds.

J wanted to know if I had a Twitter account. I did have one to promote the vacation rental but rarely used it. When Twitter first came out, I thought it was the coolest thing since sliced bread. It kept me awake at night, thinking of the possibilities. But I came to discover it is mainly used by egomaniacs and narcissists who had nothing better to do than to tweet about themselves. Can you spell brain drain? It was no more than an ego stroke. Like Ashton and Demi tweeting about their marriage. Maybe if they spoke to each other and worked on their marriage instead of tweeting about it … Is that how I REALLY felt?

J wanted me to follow Roseanne Barr. He was under the delusion that she would stop her life Monday night and help him stage a publicity stunt. Did we learn nothing from WinHawaiianHome? Thanks, Lord, for giving me a brain and enabling me to learn my lessons. Except the one that allowed me to believe he would change.

6:30 a.m., and he was using his power tools, neighbors be damned. At least he was working on his commitment instead of trying to flag down Roseanne. When I asked him if it was done, he answered, "Getting close." I rarely can get a straight answer, a yes or no. More often than not, I'd get a demeaning comment instead. He'd say things like, "I have no idea what you're talking about," or "Was there a question in there?" A few days later, at 4 a.m., he turned on the hallway light and left it on. It woke me up, putting me in a foul mood. Yet he still wondered why he couldn't get any cooperation from me.

The third annual benefit for the Puna Men's Chorus took place at the wellness retreat a mile or so down the road. J was under the delusion that they would be willing to leave their booze and pot and take a shuttle to come here and go through his HC. He actually expected people to drop their lives and plans because he snapped his fingers.

There was no map, just J's ego driving the car. A sweet old black guy came over for what he thought was supposed to be a haunted castle, and instead of working on the remodel, J spent 20 minutes showing him around. Every person that came here took him away from his focus. They stroked his ego and told him what a talented and brilliant carpenter he was, and that's what he longed for.

The broom incident: I bought a broom with a dustpan for the castle. Knowing boys will be boys and grab whatEVER WHENever, I took the broom to J and all his workers and introduced them to it. "This is MY broom for the vacation rental." I went on record so I would have something I needed where I needed it, in the pristine shape I needed it. A few days later, I went to get the broom; need I say more? He had to use MY freaking broom for HIS project, making it filthy. Was that passive-aggressive?

I will never forget the sponge incident nearly twenty years ago when we first started living together. I opened a new sponge for dishes. Typically, I took the old dish sponge and saved it for dirty jobs. J took my brand-new sponge and wiped the filthy floor. Well, back in those days, he cried that I cared more about the sponge than him. Look how far we've come.

My marriage deteriorated into Mama taking care of a two-year-old. I felt I had to take care of his body, despite his resistance, by feeding him wholesome and nourishing things so he could continue to work and get us out of the horrible financial mess. I made a salad for dinner every single day. I couldn't even put the meal out until he finished the salad because the second I did, he pushed away the salad and it was wasted unless I ate it. He wondered why his teeth were falling out. He couldn't remember to brush every day. Mama had to remind him.

J reconnected with a boyhood friend, and within months, the friend kicked him to the curb because J had yelled at him in front of people. How sad. There was an opportunity for them to work together, and for J to make decent money, but J couldn't let it happen.

One day, it was raining buckets as I was driving home, and I was joyful, gleeful even, hoping it was doing the same on our property so it would keep him inside, honoring his commitment and finishing the remodel. I was chanting: I am grateful, HappyThankYouMorePlease. That was my Mantra to Manifest.

Every chance I got, I snuck out to the trash bins to throw out some hideous crap he brought into the house without consulting me. Usually, it was something he purchased at one of those flipping auctions, and I got pleasure from doing that. That was my bad. Unacceptable by my standards. I was ashamed. I got angry at myself for sinking to his level, and then I yelled at myself for being angry in the first place. I needed to love myself. (Hear that, self?)

The Danny story: There was a young man in his early twenties, who had a small amount of cash his aunt gave him to buy some land. He also had a credit card with some credit on it. This kid didn't have a pot to p*ss in or two nickels to rub together. J got him to max his card at an auction buying materials for CIH. J promised that one day he would work off the money by helping him build something on his land. I tried to warn this guy, but he didn't listen. Now he's realizing how stupid it was because he couldn't afford freaking food and he was crying to me. I told him to talk to the hand. J's favorite saying about our community: "We are all here because we are not all there." Speak for thyself.

I had been trying for ten years to find my M&M commercial and was unsuccessful. I searched the internet, but it wasn't anywhere. Ah, the early '60s. No records. Not even the ad agency BBD&O was around anymore. My fifteen minutes. And I didn't have proof.

November 6

I got a voicemail at 12:20 a.m. "Aloha, I'm driving home on the Keaau bypass road, and I think the driver of your van, which is clearly labeled "CastleinHawaii," is very drunk. Whoever is driving can't keep himself on the road. I saw him cut across two lanes of traffic to get on the bypass road, so I wanted you to be aware of that. I'm following him now, but I hope you don't let this person drive inebriated again. All right, have a good evening. Aloha."

November 7

Ruth and Leo arrived, and we gave them a tour so they could get familiar with the area. Once they settled in, I cooked for them, and we spent time getting to know each other.

There was nothing like waking up to being called "stupid" first thing in the morning and then the "c" word. Why didn't he just put them both together and call me "stupid c*t" to save himself some time? He did it in front of Ruth; she was not amused, and I was embarrassed.

I was so tired of owing money to friends, family, and neighbors. Now came the topper. Instead of doing what he was supposed to do for the remodel, he grabbed Leo, and they went to an auction. I warned Leo that we had no money to buy anything and had tons of credit card debt.

Sure as hell, they came home with a truck-load of garbage and spent almost $600, which he got Leo to put on his card. Well, he couldn't say I didn't warn him. I tried to impress on J that we needed to get the cards down. That didn't exist on Planet J. He came home with a gift for me. A huge, hideous Christmas snow globe. He told me, "This will be worth something in five or ten years." I doubted it. I have a snow globe collection of about twenty-plus globes. Mine were exquisite, over fifty years old and were already worth something.

November 8

At 4 a.m., the fun started again. He was up, doing who knows what, and woke me. When I went into my office, I found him running around naked. Was that a clue? He was near my computer, which I always made sure to turn off at the end of the day, but it was on. When I asked why he was on my computer, he casually said, "I wanted to print something." Well, usually the secretary—that would be me—printed things. I didn't want him near my desk. I went to the computer and said, "Tell me what you want to print, and I'll do it." On the browser, I saw: FREE PORN. Why was I constantly surprised?

November 9

I felt like I'd been waterboarded. I could barely keep my eyes open. J had worked from midnight till 6 a.m., stomping around in work boots so I was awake pretty much all night. I thought we lived in Hawaii, where everyone takes off their shoes indoors.

He was supposed to be Santa at the mall starting November 18th for six weeks for $25/hr. It's better than a poke in the eye with a sharp stick. Now, he was injecting a Ren Faire in the park into his schedule, even though we had guests. Even though no one in the community wanted or supported this. A Renaissance or Medieval fair was an outdoor gathering aimed at recreating a historical setting. He informed me that when he worked as Santa, he would change the direct deposit, take the money, and not pay the credit cards down as he promised. I told him if he did that, then I'd make sure he didn't get that job. I'd call the lady and mention his proclivity to surf "free porn." He said he'd been doing porn since we stopped having sex however many years ago, which meant he went to the temple with a temple recommend on a lie. In the Church of Jesus Christ of Latter-day Saints, a member has to affirm their honesty, moral cleanliness, adherence to church teachings, and willingness to keep sacred covenants to enter the temple. It was just one more area in his life where he was not being honest or taking responsibility. I no longer knew the man I married twenty years ago.

He didn't want to admit his part in the mess we were calling our lives. Live alone, die alone. I was very alone. I planned to carry my iPhone and tape these conversations from then on. How sad that this was how I had to conduct my life. He left the door to the Echo open, and it started to pour. When I told him the inside of the car was getting soaked, he said, "That sucks."

November 10

One evening, working in my office, I was enjoying the roar of the coqui frogs. They might sound like crickets, but they say, "Coqui, Coqui" almost deafeningly. They were accidentally introduced to the Big Island in the late 80s on imported plants from Puerto Rico. They lack natural predators that keep their population down.

J came in and complained that my office smelled like an ashtray. If that's what it took to keep him out, then I'd smoke there. I had been smoking outside. My lungs hurt. I knew I needed to quit again. I hated how I'd been so good at not smoking since June, even spending $150 on Chantix for a month. What a complete waste. I had a love/hate relationship with that drug, and it's only meant to be used once, but I could already predict I'd be turning to it again soon.

What straw broke the camel's back? It was the "mine" issue. I touched a tool, and he said, "That's mine." He tried to take my laptop with him when he left, and I said, "That's mine." So, he flung it. I called the Bishop after the incident, and he told me, "Stay safe, and if you have to call the authorities, do so." I called J and told him the Bishop's advice, and he said, "Do what you have to do." I said, "No, I'll do what you force me to do."

Ruth and Leo told me that cars were stopping in front of the house to hear the ruckus of our continual fights. OMG, this was the reputation he wanted us to have in our community? This is what he wanted to be known for? It was mortifying.

There is a saying: charity begins at home. His charity and just about anything and everything else was more important to him than us and our home. I discovered that he got Wally World to increase his card's limit from $300 to $900, and he had already maxed that out in a couple of weeks. Then he demanded I pay it off. So he can just blow it on his new venture? Renaissance Fair in the park. I think it's scheduled for November 26th, not sure since he didn't tell me.

When I asked him to leave the house, he said, "I'm not leaving *my* house." The last time I looked, it was *our* house. I reached out to his brother and sister on the mainland and begged them to help and come up with an answer. Then I called Lynette and told her how lucky she was. She agreed and was empathetic, since she had been married to him. They all told me what an a*hole he was at Jessie's funeral, the young niece he adored. They thought he was insane. When I told him what they said, his answer was, "I AM insane." Yup, can I hear an amen? He was telling inappropriate jokes or something at his beloved young niece's memorial.

I needed to get a lock for my office. If he broke my desktop computer, I would be unable to work my ass into an early grave to try to stay afloat. I didn't know how to play chess, but I felt like I had to play the game of my life. Stay one step ahead so he doesn't hurt me. He accused me of listening when he was on the phone, so I guess that's his justification when I caught him listening to my conversations. Smoking myself to death just like my dad. Resentments cause cancer, no?

November 10

J and I were arguing about something. He erupted in a violent outburst, hurling my laptop and a brand-new computer monitor across the room. The scene was a haunting echo of his behavior in Fullerton, triggering déjà vu. I told him he had to leave - just as I had before. I packed his bag.

Hours later, he returned to collect his belongings. This time, Ruth was there to ensure he didn't lose control again. When he got there, I said, "I think I remembered everything." He grabbed the bag, looked in it, and asked, "Did you pack my iPhone charger?" I said, "No, I guess I didn't remember everything, sue me," and he said, "That's next." Another threat. I should have been used to it by then.

I found the motion lotion he had dropped in the file box under my desk he used for his porn sessions, so I packed that for him too! I also found condoms in his pocket. Apparently, he hadn't just been surfing for free porn.

After he left, I smoked what I had hoped would be my "last" cig, took a valerian, a tryptophan, and a melatonin. I set the sleep timer and slept fitfully until morning.

At 2 a.m., I woke up for my first pee break. I think the bladder thing had a lot to do with the stress and anxiety, so I tried to power through, squeezing my eyes shut. The second one was at 4 a.m., and I took another tryptophan. At least I didn't drink a bottle of wine or even a sip! But I will admit that I wanted a cig, and I wanted one bad. Ruth told me she had quit and to take one day at a time. I knew that unless he seeks therapy and treatment, nothing will change. No wonder most women didn't leave; it was too hard. It was easier to just stay and take it.

November 11

I decided to have the castle blessing since it was all planned. J came to help get the place ready. He was supposed to take the dining table from our house on the second floor to the CH house. In the middle of taking off the legs so he could move it, he walked away and said, "You f*cking do it," in front of my girlfriend who was helping me. He also threatened, "You'll see tomorrow who everything belongs to."

Later in the day, he came back and demanded some receipts I had of his. They were actually tickets for a concert he was going to see, which I didn't notice. I had been asking for Nat's wedding band back from him for days. I sensed this was my chance to get it and told him if he wanted the tickets, he had to give me back my dad's wedding band. He flung it at me. I put it on. I'm sure Nat was rolling over in his grave. At least the ring was on MY finger where it belonged. I'd always worn his wife's (matching) band. Now they were no longer a symbol of my marriage but rather a connection to my dead dad. I had made a Gourmet Catering ring with our GC logo and he threw it into the lava.

I woke up at 3:30 a.m. I jumped onto Facebook, and Laura in NY, who was six hours ahead, was on, so we messaged back and forth for a few minutes. As usual, she supported and comforted me and urged me to try and go back to sleep. I took a tryptophan, and thankfully, one of them didn't make me too groggy to function the following morning. I must stick to my guns and get some good karma going. We both needed help, but I would resolve to keep trying to help myself. I didn't want the wrath of the karma gods. I had to live an authentic life with intention. Wish me luck. We waited so long and worked so hard to be finished, so we could move from the CH to the second and third floors of the main house, which was our apartment. Now that that has happened, we have separated. Why must things end like this?

November 13

The blessing was incredible—spiritual and uplifting. I had someone record it, but unfortunately, the quality of the video was less than ideal. Still, I believe it cleared away all the bad energy and negative juju. We (the royal "we") were already feeling stronger, although still somewhat depressed.

I wrote him and asked him to write back:

Dear J,

Since we don't seem to be able to speak, I am writing you. I found this online: "Contacting a mediator, lawyer, or other professional to help you resolve your issues is necessary, but give yourself at least a couple of weeks or a month. Unless there is some alarming movement of money, keeping things status quo for 30 days is not going to make a difference in the long term. Request that things remain status quo until you can both start laying the foundation and making sound decisions about how you are going to move forward. The fear is when one party feels that the other party has had a massive head start and perhaps got their ducks in a row long before informing their spouse of their intentions. That may be the case, but that is water under the bridge right now."

Can you tell me what you want? You wrote your ex … maybe you can write me. If you care what I want, and I know you always say you do not, here it is anyway:

1. Peace and space for the next month while you are being Santa. And if you want or need to come onto the property, the courtesy of a phone call to let me know.

2. I'd like to know your intentions about contributing to our massive bills with the pay you will be getting for the Santa gig. You indicated you were just going to keep this money and let me "deal" with everything. Is this so? Sounds like our catering company all over again. I'm not out to hurt you. We should work together so both of us do not get hurt financially or physically. I cannot predict if we can heal emotionally. Time will tell. I attached a list of what is due right now, it totals approximately $4,000.

3. Spend a peaceful hour together daily to watch the Oprah Life Classes. "Love does not hurt," so sayeth Oprah. Hurtful words are just that, hurtful. You can't unring a bell.

4. Indicate that you are willing to put our healing before all your other activities.

5. I need to quit cigs, and I need your help and support, not your derision, criticism, and judgment.

I can't understand why it seems that every ten years, things go haywire with you. I must remind you that ten years ago, you apologized and promised that "things would be different" and asked me to come to Hawaii to heal. Was that all just a ruse to sell our house and put everything in your dad's name? This last year was no different than 2000.

When I tried to hand him the letter, he asked, "Are you serving me?" Had he never heard the third-party rule? A person cannot serve their opponent; a third party has to do it. That's what I have to deal with. Everything was competitive and a struggle just to have a civil conversation. I heard from Legal Aid and the attorney said he wasn't sure if he could take the case as they didn't usually allow self-employed people to get aid. I was in tears, begging him. Hopefully I'll know shortly. If not, I'm screwed.

I couldn't believe what happened. Ruth and I were getting ready to go out. When I came downstairs, Ruth said, "J was here; he took some lettuce to the park."Me: "Lettuce? I don't have any lettuce." I looked in the fridge, and all my food was gone. I gave J most of the leftovers from the blessing yesterday, so I was confused. I kept the vegetable crudité and some mac salad. I thought I'd make a huge comforting pot of veggie soup, try to coax myself to eat, and freeze the rest. I ran outside, and J was in the Echo, starting to drive out of the community. I opened the passenger door to prevent him from leaving and to speak to me.

Me: "Where is all my food?"

J: "I gave it to the hippies in the park."

Me: "Why did you do that?"

J: "They needed food."

Me: "I need food! Would you be willing to not take anything from the property without telling or asking me?

J: "No."

The mac salad was in my favorite Tupperware. Anyone who knew me knew I was very anal about my Tupperware. I was almost in tears at this point. I told him I had no money for food and asked why he would give all my food away. No answer. I went out to the park to the picnickers and told them, "J stole my food; food that I need to live on since he maxed out all my credit cards, and I can't afford to pay bills or buy food." Well, of course, they gave me back my stuff.

Ruth kept shaking her head; she couldn't believe what she saw. She confided that they were relieved he wasn't there anymore. Why was he acting this way? Did he think there were no repercussions for his actions? He was forcing me to get a restraining order so he could blame everything on me. God, please let me manifest an attorney, I beg you. I need help; I need protection.

November 14

At 6 a.m., I got up to get ready to go to court. I had to leave by 8 a.m. to try to get a TRO (temporary restraining order). I was terrified to leave, lest things went missing. Ruth said she and Leo would stay, but I knew there would be very little they could do if he decided to make drama.

When I got back, I sat in my office, working and enjoying the peace. I heard J pull up. I went down to see why he was there. I asked him, "Why can't you call before you come?" J: "I don't want to." The reason he came, as far as I could tell, was to bring his dirty laundry for me to do. I would do it with the intention of keeping him out of here. If I couldn't do it with love, I wouldn't do it. I asked him yet again if he could possibly be willing to respect my wishes. His answer again was no.

November 16

I know I was a glutton for punishment and asked him: "J, can you agree to the following? Until your answer is yes, it will be very difficult to proceed."

1. If you want or need to come onto the property, the courtesy of a phone call to let me know. I want someone to be with me when you are here.

2. Your word that you WILL NOT come on the property when no one is here and/or take stuff from here without telling me what you need or will be taking. ESPECIALLY food. It's not like I don't share what I have.

3. I'd like to know your intentions about contributing to our massive bills with the pay you will be getting for the Santa gig.

4. Create a schedule for Bruiser, including when you will drop him off each day and when you will pick him up.

5. Drop off your laundry on Friday. I will try to turn it around in 24 hours.

This was his reply:

"FORECASTING THE FUTURE! (Formalized Madness) All that I have created physically is yours. Just allow me enough time before you completely abandon our spiritual bond. You can have the stuff; just let me finish my destiny. Time grows short. How much do you have left? Stop telling people I'm insane; it reflects badly on you. Besides, what is madness? Maybe too much sanity is madness, but the maddest of all is 'seeing the world as it is and not as it should be' (Don Quixote). I thought that you valued truth above all else. I guess I was wrong … again."

The next day, he came, gave me his receipts, and told me, "I'm taking my tools to hock them for my legal bills." Legal bills for the spec house? Trying to rectify the foreclosure? He took the wet-dry vac, air compressor, and table saw. I asked why he had the van and trailer to go to court. "I'm working for Habitat for Humanity today." I thought to myself, but they don't PAY you.

The judge granted my request for a temporary restraining order. I believed J needed psychiatric help. And if he needed it and did not get it, then what? My brain was spinning.

At 3 p.m., he delivered this letter:

Sheri,

I do not fear life anymore. You must have seen this conflict coming because how else will we learn? I saw Jessie in her coffin, the purest soul I have ever known. No one knows when their time is finished, so why fear time or waste it? There is only one pursuit of any worth, and that is service to my fellow men and women, no matter who or what they are. The proof is there every minute that shows me that my actions are right.

You must provide me with opposition until the truth prevails and we can no longer hide our true selves behind the facade of the world. I know I am different. I have no shame in being different; I will make a difference in this world, and you will help me by hurting me, but it's ok. You must follow your path also. We cannot change one another, only our destiny in this world.

All I could think of was that it was too bad his service didn't include his wife and home, and he didn't answer or address a single issue in my letter to him. No surprise.

November 17

We had no water. J came over and agreed to install the water pump and pressure tank so we could have water. Then he said he needed to eat breakfast first, so I gave him a bowl of cereal. Then it started.

J: "How much will you pay me to install the water pump?"

Me: "How about if I fill up the Echo so you can meet your commitment and start the Santa gig on Saturday?"

J: "Fill up the van too."

Me: "I don't have a hundred dollars to fill up that gas guzzler to pay for your charity."

He called me the "c" word in front of Ruth again. I couldn't wait until they served the TRO. I then knew the meaning of the phrase irreconcilable differences. I said black; he said white. I know that God doesn't give us what we cannot bear. I knew I would get through this, but at what expense? Not eating, not sleeping?

November 20

He dropped Bruiser off at 8:30 a.m., and I had the most peaceful, blissful day. I set another quit date for Monday. I must be strong. I actually slept last night. I was able to eat some healthy things today; what more could a girl ask for? For the first time in twenty years, I finally got to do what I wanted. If he worked from 10 a.m. to 8 p.m., I guessed he would pick Bruiser up at 9ish.

November 21

I went to the mall to try to find the Echo while he was working so I could fill it up, so he had no excuse not to go to his gig. I found it following my intuition. The key was in the ignition, all the doors were unlocked, and all his crap was every-where. I went to turn on the ignition to see how much gas was in the tank, and the car was dead. So I left. I wondered why I even went there and wasted my time. A little later, a friend called and asked why my car was in the parking lot with all the windows open in the pouring rain. Who knows why anything anymore?

November 25, Thanksgiving

J and a few of his buddies came to the property to set up his Ren Faire. Ruth and Leo called the police. They came, they arrested him, they took him to jail. What a great way to spend the holiday. I had the guys who were helping him set up tear it all down.

November 27

I wrote him:

> J, at the risk of repeating myself:
>
> I am not out to hurt you or be mean and vindictive as you seem to believe. Why do you have to do this and then say, "It's something that had to be done." It doesn't have to be done. Do you like hitting rock bottom? Going to jail is fun? Or are you just trying to prove you are above the law? What good can come of alienating your neighbors and great community (your words) in your flyer campaigning for support for the Ren Faire?
>
> It sounds like 1999 when I was left with the three-and-a-half-million-dollar sinking ship. If you were going to change the direct deposit for the Santa gig, why on earth would I care if you got arrested?

You were willing to take off for your sweetheart cottage court date but not for your marriage or to spare yourself from going to jail—your choices, no? You might want to reexamine your priorities.

Let me be crystal clear. Our neighbors are aware of the TRO. You might be turned in by someone other than me. Do I still get blamed? In fact, I was admonished by a couple of them that I should have called the police already. Actually, Ruth said she would call the next time you come here, she's had enough. Frankly, I don't blame her. How dare you wake them up at 5:30 in the morning? Did you really think that would be ok? This was NOT what they signed up for when they gave us four months rent in advance to finish the remodel.

I will protect our vacation rental business from you at all costs. I haven't worked these past ten years to flush it, even if you are willing to do so. Have it your way; you are taking all the actions. I was just here minding my own beeswax, trying to have some peace in my life after twenty-one years. If you bring people onto the property on Saturday like you said you were going to, you will have to pay the consequences. Bishop sent you a letter just like the one you got from your Bishop in Fullerton in 1999. Why can't you learn from your past actions? Why do you need to repeat them over and over?

This is what I got back from J:

You already know how this game ends, so why keep playing it? Just as you feel you must follow your own path, so must I. This game has no winners, only losers. I do not fear anything. I laid Jessie in her grave; we all will soon follow. Is this how you want to end the game? Money will not buy you life; it will only diminish it. I gave you my heart, and you consistently and methodically torture it. Thank you, I need this. It's all just dust, but you know this, don't you? I am going to have to stop my pay from going to you. How else can I survive? If you have me arrested, my contract as Santa will be canceled. And contractually, I will lose all I have earned thus far.

ALTERNATE REALITY:

You stop trying to destroy me and my relationships with others. You stop trying to ruin my charity fundraiser and help me instead.

You allow me to follow my path before my death.

You love me by transcending your reality.

You accept my love by not judging me.

You love yourself by seeing that we are one.

We make our reality; we choose our destiny.

(signed) one who knows

December 1

I was on my way to Hilo for the hearing, or whatever it was, for the spec house since J was incarcerated, I thought I should make an appearance.

Saturday, two guys who worked on the Haunted Castle with J stopped by to lend support. QB is a sweet guy, and DB is a firefighter/boxer. I'd only met them once on Halloween. They seemed nice, but I hadn't seen them since then. DB said J seemed to jump off the deep end in front of their very eyes.

Days later, J was out in front of the house in a car with a woman. At some point, he climbed over the queen lanai, and I blew. "What the hell are you doing? I have guests!" I didn't, but I could have. He mumbled an apology and I told him in no uncertain terms that he was not to come on this property. He can ring the bell, and I will come out. I demanded the book he took from one of the suites, *Big Island Revealed*. I kept one in every rental space for the guests. He said he left it somewhere.

After he left, I approached the woman who had brought him who was still sitting in her car in the park. She said they were at ecstatic dance, and she was forced to do the community a service by removing him since he couldn't shut up. Ecstatic dance is a free-form, unstructured dance inspired and led by carefully crafted music with the intention of creating a healing journey. No dance experience or partner is necessary or needed. All in silence.

A neighbor called and told me that apparently J went to Uncle Robert's open-air farmer's market and was asking for free fruit. The girl there said he made her very uncomfortable. Then I got a call from another neighbor who said some lady in the community picked him up hitchhiking, and he seemed like he was trying to steal her phone. He told all these people that he was staying at the castle. I told them that was a lie. I think about an Oprah show I saw, and her guest said, "If you see crazy coming, cross the street!"

He got arrested again and was incarcerated. The judge ordered a psych evaluation. If the court system takes the spec house, I feared it would push him over the edge. Oops, I think that has already happened. Another mess to clean up. I was so conflicted. I don't really understand his mental illness, but I meant to find out the results of the psych eval.

Sunday, I went to church to get some ward love, and see Bishop. When I saw the woman who sold us Bruiser, I sat next to her. Something clicked in my brain that she worked for the system, but I didn't remember in what capacity. She was the one who called me about the Echo in the rain. Then I remembered she worked at the jail in Hilo. She told me she was there when J was brought in. I pumped her for info, but she didn't or perhaps couldn't share much (standard operating procedure for the legal system).

December 10

J had Daniel, our architect, draw up plans for the courtyard. I never knew J asked him to do it. And I never got to see it. All I knew about the plans was that there was another kitchen. OH, HELL NO. We needed another kitchen (there are three here already), like we needed another orifice in the cabeza (hole in the head).

My life read like a poorly written comedy. Tripping over things, falling down, hurting myself by accident, distracted to the max. Trying to do things in a rush. I got a hysterical back, which is what I called my flare-ups of sciatica. It only seemed to appear at times of extreme stress. All the phone lines were ringing at once. All kinds of court dates to remember and keep track of. Things going on with this house … stuff falling off in my hands, water suddenly stopped working. I had to reset the circuit breakers. There were things J promised to do or fix that were not done. It seemed like everything I touched did not work properly, or you had to be a rocket scientist to figure out how it worked. You couldn't just turn the hot tub on. J configured this like everything else in this house in a complicated, convoluted way. If it wasn't so sad, it would have been funny. If you don't laugh, you cry. I questioned my Karma; it needed repair. I thought I broke my husband; I must have also broken my Karma.

I had gone to the Pahoa police station to make a report about his coming onto the property. The officer suggested a TRO as he left to do the paperwork. I had one of those, and it wasn't doing anything for my situation. The officer then told me, "Never mind, just call 911, and we'll pick him up." Huh? Apparently there was a warrant out for his arrest, but they wouldn't tell me what it was for. Typical police method of operation. A sad statement for Hawaii … but typical.

At 3 a.m., I bolted upright in bed. I thought I heard "hello," but I must have been dreaming. Boy, did I want motion detector lights, then I could have security AND conserve AND be in alignment with my community. If you didn't keep lights off at night, the neighborhood pitched a fit. This was for the observatory and the stars. When I finally got up in the morning, my back seized. I couldn't move; I couldn't even breathe.

2012

January 22

The pool pump wouldn't stop running. It overflowed into the park sending our electric bills sky-high. Every time it kicked on, I knew it was costing big bucks, and I felt the weight of it all. Despite having solar, the bills were staggering—$600 in November, $800 in December. How could this be happening? I felt overwhelmed, drowning in frustration with costs I couldn't control. How the hell was this happening?

I suspected the well pump had been running nonstop for a month. Most people here used catchment systems, but not J. No, he had to have a well—just 300 yards from the ocean. Everyone knew drilling that close to the ocean was a terrible idea. Everyone except J, of course.

I went to court to make the TRO permanent. My options?

1. Drop it, which J asked me to do as it was "frivolous," according to him

2. Keep it, which entailed returning for an evidentiary hearing where evidence was produced to make the order of protection permanent. This meant more court dates, then, it would become a restraining order.

3. Make it a "full contact" order of protection—basically, the judge telling him to behave like a decent human being. As if that would work.

4. These people had no clue. None at all.

I was pissed at myself. Still smoking, hating every damn cigarette. No exercise. No movement. A total slug. No motivation. No joy.

Still, I had to be grateful. Every time someone booked a suite, I thanked God. Grateful for my health and Ray. I had prayed for a miracle for him and got it! He was doing so well that I kept pinching myself. Had I imagined that horrible week of agony a few years back?

Tax time. Another $2,000 due. Another prayer for a miracle. Enough to fix things. Enough to finish this place. But should I even stay? If I walked away … where would I go? What the hell would I do?

This was my passion—to be an innkeeper, share Hawaiian culture, and coordinate destination weddings. Especially cooking for people. When I cooked, I created and let out my inner artist. I got pleasure from seeing people enjoy what I created. Wishing there was a grant or something I could get. I had an idea that I could give the suites to Make-a-Wish. Kids could be a King or Queen to forget whatever they were going through with their illness.

February 1

I woke up at 5, went to the bathroom, and somehow managed to fall back asleep until just before 6. I made coffee and crawled back into bed, and listened to my stop-smoking hypnosis tape. After getting dressed, I headed downstairs for more coffee, gave Ray his pills, and took his meat for the day out of the freezer to defrost. Then Ray and I went for our usual 45-minute walk, ending at the cliff. We stood there together, watching the waves crash against the shore. As I poured out my heart to him, he looked into my eyes with such deep compassion—listening the way only he could. Like he was desperately trying to understand my words. I couldn't love anyone more than I loved this boy. More than life itself.

Leo had been sick the past week. We thought it was a virus or flu. Ruth was going to Kona, and when she went to say goodbye to him and found him unresponsive. She took him to the hospital and discovered he had been drinking rum for days. She found two empty bottles under their sink.

After three days of intensive care, he came home. Dear Lord, I pray for them. We all have problems, just different problems. They have all the money they need but not happiness. Addiction sucks. Tobacco was mine, and alcohol was Leo's. Some may have one; some may have both. No one ever said life would be easy. And what doesn't kill you makes you stronger, right? I'll let ya know.

Yesterday, J came and took something. It wasn't about what he took but the fact that he came on the property. This wasn't the first time. I tried to be calm and rational, but he was so irrational it's difficult to take a higher road.

I went to a hula lesson. I didn't participate, though. Sometimes I feel shy, and I wasn't sure if I could do it, so I just watched. But something stirred in me, and I thought, maybe next week I'd give it a whirl. I just felt uncoordinated and the idea of dancing in front of people now, as an adult, made me sweat. It's not like when I was seven and fearless.

February 16

4:30 a.m. Awake. Weeping. Yesterday, J hit a new low. He was out in the park in front of the house, wearing that damn Santa hat, so I went down to check on Bruiser and get a little puppy love. I hadn't seen him since J left for his camping trip to Plastic Beach. Kamilo Beach was one of the dirtiest beaches in the world, strewn with plastic so people here call it Plastic Beach for a good reason. This little sausage had eaten raw meat for 99% of his life, and I had no idea what he had been fed since J took him. I couldn't shake the thought that the group of hippies they were with might be vegan. I imagined this poor wiener being offered just fruit and veggies. Now J was using him as a pawn and wouldn't let me love on him.

The bank had obtained a summary judgment for the SC, meaning they won the case and got the house, along with a writ of possession granting them the authority to have a sheriff physically remove J and anyone else inside, along with all possessions in the house. The judge had given him until February 17 to find a new place to live. His dad and wife wrote me an email expressing their support for this decision. Well, she wrote it; he couldn't read or write.

I went to the SC to ask when he was moving out. Where was he going? What was his plan? When I got there, I walked straight into a sea of humanity. He had filled the house with anyone wanting to crash. Can you spell flop house? J was sitting in the driveway with a group of twenty to thirty kids forming a semi-circle in front of him, hanging on his every word. He was in his element, soaking up the attention. Or perhaps he was forming a cult.

After twenty-two years, I had no idea who this man was anymore. He was Mormon, then he wasn't. He never smoked, then he was a potaholic, and all he did was smoke. He never lied or manipulated; now, he was proud he had become a master of both. He stole—well, from me, anyway. He came to the house and shopped, as my girlfriend put it.

After his sermon, we went inside the house, and I asked if he had seen the email. He claimed he hadn't. When I delivered it, I placed it on the counter. I opened a drawer, found it, and handed it to him, but he tried to put it back. I took it from him and read it aloud. "I'm not leaving," he snapped. "Don't touch anything."

What J was doing with his life, in my opinion, was just so wrong. Is this a textbook midlife crisis? Or is it a mental defect—ADHD, Messiah complex, narcissism, bipolar? And why did I feel the need to put a label on it? I guess because I wondered how you could fix something if you didn't know what it was.

Someone told me a funny story. Once upon a time, there was a woman who loved to fish. She was sitting in her boat fishing when she heard a voice say, "Pick me up." She looked around and couldn't see anyone. She thought she was dreaming when she heard the voice say again, "Pick me up."

She looked in the water, and there, floating on the top, was a frog. The woman asked, "Are you talking to me?" The frog said, "Yes, I'm talking to you. Pick me up, kiss me, and I'll turn into the most handsome man you have ever seen. I'll make sure that all your friends are jealous because I will be your groom!"

The woman looked at the frog for a short time, reached over, picked it up, and placed it in her shirt pocket. The frog said, "Are you nuts? Didn't you hear what I said? She opened her pocket, looked at the frog, and said, "Nah. I'd rather have a talking frog."

I felt so empty inside. Life barely felt like living. I had to keep reminding myself of my blessings and count them one by one. That was from a song we sang at church. Bishop called J and asked him to go see a therapist. I doubted he would do that. I was lonely. There were people around me, but I was lonely. OK, enough self-pity.

February 18

I decided to write to my Mom. This is the letter that I had longed to write to her.

I wrote it to vent, but I never sent it. (Smart girl.)

Aloha Mama, Mom, Mother, Mommy,

I've had this burning need to communicate with you. To say what? I love you? I miss you? Yes AND mainly to say I'm sorry I was never the daughter you hoped for. I see other people who have a great mother-daughter relationship, and my heart aches, and my emotions go from longing to "Is that for real"?

Most mothers are loving, forgiving, and long-suffering, for good or bad. Isn't that what God intended? Not critical and unforgiving like you have been. My most vivid memory of you is when you and George searched my room and read my mail. That invasion of privacy shaped my life.

Birthday cards had to get to you before your birthday. If I sent you a birthday card and it didn't arrive before the date, look out. If I parted my hair, you thought it would be better pulled back in a ponytail and made sure I knew it.

I guess in your eyes, I've always been a disappointment. I accept this for what it is. When I win the lottery, I intend to pay off your house anonymously. Just because. Seems like all you ever cared about is money or a lack of it.

I've asked you on numerous occasions to come here and see what we built, to see our castle. You never had the time or the inclination to do so. It made me sad. I have an email that you sent me with venomous comments about your reverse mortgage and how I should stop wishing for your death so I would inherit your house. Really? I have never asked for anything. During all the years I was growing up, you and George were the ones who kept telling me, in case of your death, to go here and find this, go there and find that. Here's a key for the safe and the safety deposit box at the bank. You wrote a note listing your assets. At the time, I was touched and honored, but, in the end, when George passed, I got nada, which is fine. I have never thought about what you were going to leave me or what I would get after you were gone.

I wondered, was this a carrot you dangled for your love? Then, if I didn't act like you wanted me to, you would take it away with your love. I don't blame you because I know your mother shaped who you are and showered her love and support on Aunt Sheila.

Maybe I should never have written this, but at least I'm smart enough not to send it. I pray for Ho'oponopono (Hawaiian healing). I love you; I miss you. You're my mama.

Aloha, Your daughter

March 1

I was sitting in my office when I heard clanging. Peering out the window, I saw J wheeling away one of our huge propane tanks on our dolly. I had just filled it with $100 worth of propane. It was also our newest tank. He was leaving the property with it. I raced down three flights of stairs. I confronted him and demanded to know what he was doing. No answer, as if I really expected one. He was stealing it. Duh.

I raced back up to my office, grabbed my iPhone so I could take pictures to document this incident, jumped in the car, and sped up Mapuana, the main road of the subdivision. I found him putting the tank into a silver Chevy PT Cruiser with a girl I recognized from the flop house. I took a picture of her license plate and of him loading the tank into her car. He left the dolly in the middle of the street. I retrieved it and stashed it in my car, then returned home and called the police. They said there was nothing they could do.

I called Turning Point, who had prepared the paperwork for the TRO. I requested that they modify the "full contact" TRO to a "no contact" TRO. However, it turned out that after they served him, she didn't ask them to expedite it, and it was scheduled for April 17! I knew I wouldn't last until then.

March 7

Leslie was staying with me, keeping me company, and would be at the castle to take care of guests and business when I went to the mainland. Sometime after 7 or 8 p.m., her boyfriend, Ben, called. He said that he had a call from the security guards where he lived at the entrance of the lava flow. J was at the gate making a scene and almost got into a fistfight with the guard. No cars were supposed to pass, except for residents. Many tourists came wanting to walk on the flow, so the county made them park and walk. J told security that Ben expected him and that he had something very important to discuss with him. Ben told the guard he wasn't expecting J and had nothing to discuss with him. Somehow, J managed to talk his way in, he got to Ben's house, and started to babble about "occupy" or some such nonsense.

March 12

I was in Cali for my yearly trip, and Leslie was at the house. I went to the NPE (Natural Product Expo) to see what was new in health. Every year I got an abundance of samples that usually lasted a year or more. I got my teeth cleaned, went to the dermatologist for a skin checkup, got a mammography, saw my primary for a yearly wellness checkup and got a blood test, etc. I've been seeing my docs for over twenty-five years. I wasn't about to change at this stage of my life.

J came to the house at 4:30 a.m. Leslie was there with Ben. She immediately called me, when she heard someone walking around my bedroom on the third floor. They were sleeping on the second floor on the couch in the living room. J had climbed up outside to the third floor and came into the bedroom, which did not have a lock. He has said, on several occasions, that he could get in the house any time he pleased since he built the place. J then came downstairs and started harassing them.

March 13

I landed in Honolulu at 1:30 p.m and got a call from Carol, my neighbor in the house right behind the castle, who said there were about ten to twenty people all over the castle, drinking and smoking and having a great party. I called the police.

The day before, J had called me and asked to come over to do laundry. I told him to wait until the next day, and I would do it. I was hoping he didn't know I was in California. I was an idiot to think that.

When the police came, all the partyers had disappeared, and J told them he was there to do laundry. They left because there was nothing they could do. I called Turning Point and asked them to expedite the "no contact" TRO. She told me to come in and sign the paperwork when I landed in Hilo.

I did.

When I finally got home from Hilo at 6 p.m., I went to my office, where the laundry room is located and is always kept locked, to find the door broken and piles of filthy, stinky laundry all over my office floor and the laundry room floor. The door can't close now, which means when it rains, the rain will come into the room.

I found a carving on the bedroom door. I also noticed that there were missing screws on all the doors. I would have to replace every freaking door with non removable pins if I were ever to feel secure in this place.

I took pictures with my iPhone. I gathered all the laundry and deposited it on the street. Then I drove to the SC—which I now called the flop house. He was not there. A girl there called me a bitch when I told her the laundry was on the street. I left, and soon after, three men in a small burgundy Nissan came and picked up all the laundry and tried to take Bruiser, who was with me. I grabbed the dog and told them, "No freaking way." I probably used the other word; I was so angry. I took pictures of them, the car, and the license plate.

Our vacation rental guests from Texas said their room looked rifled through. A bottle of rum that had been on the lanai table and some beers from their fridge were missing. Her purse with her credit cards was in one of the drawers. They said they didn't think any were taken, but they were worried that maybe someone copied the numbers. There was also an empty orange juice container on the breezeway counter that had not been there when they left. J had helped himself to my fridge. There were two one-hundred-dollar bills in a drawer on the second floor, which was their security deposit, and I was to return them when they left. It was gone.

Ruth and Leo were supposed to be here until May 1, but they have given me notice that they cannot take any more drama with J's behavior. We were losing a month's income.

I wrote the judge a letter detailing the events above and closed the letter:

Judge, if this isn't harassment and a violation of the full contact TRO, then I don't know what is. He is disrupting our business and will destroy it if he is not stopped. He has no respect for the law. I believe he is mentally unstable. People told me he is drinking alcohol, which he never did before in our 22 years of marriage. He told me he had been smoking pot. He admits he is a potaholic, and smoking makes him nuts. He has told me in no uncertain terms that he can come into the house at any time and take anything he pleases. He built the place, and nothing and no one could keep him from getting in. His erratic behavior is terrifying. My doctor has prescribed anti-anxiety and anti-depression drugs for me, which I am reluctant to take because I don't like taking meds. He has made my life a living hell, and I would be grateful for relief from the court.

I am urgently requesting that you grant a no-contact TRO and forbid him from coming to the Castle and destroying the business we have been building for the last four years. He had been ordered for psych eval by the court due to his increasingly erratic behavior, and I hope you agree his actions justify this protection. His continued presence puts me, and everything we've built, at serious risk. I am now paying the physical and emotional price.

March 14, J's Birthday

Earlier today, I saw J pass by squashed in the back of a pickup truck with a bunch of hippies, wearing that ridiculous Santa hat again. I had the overwhelming urge to burn that hat. He actually wore that hat to court once. The judge asked him to take it off, and he flat-out refused. His other court "uniform" was a Boy Scout shirt, sometimes paired with an African beanie. Does that sound like mental competence?

Another example of J's instability was at Puna's funeral. Puna, Uncle Robert's son, died suddenly at age 44 of a heart attack. As strange as it sounds, I felt a pang of envy. Good for Puna, he was in a better place. How I wished that were me. J showed up to the Celebration of Life at Uncle Robert's in his Boy Scout shirt carrying his briefcase. There were hundreds of people there, all dressed appropriately for the occasion, and not a single briefcase in sight—except for his. Yet another reminder of how out of touch he was with reality.

I was parking the Echo and the Rav behind my house. Not that he wouldn't be able to see them, I was just hoping he wouldn't. I wanted him to think I wasn't home, hoping to catch him trying to break in again. The sad part? This is what my life had come to—living in constant fear, protecting myself from my own husband. It was pathetic, and yet, somehow, this was my new normal. Pathetic.

The judge denied my request to revise the TRO. (Insert sarcastic *YAY* here.) Looks like it's time to lawyer up. I found an attorney who was supposed to call me and let me know what it would cost to get the TRO. He was a criminal attorney, which was not really what I needed, but there were slim pickings around here. I just hoped he knew what he was doing. Spoiler alert: he didn't. Years later, I got a letter from the Hawaii Disciplinary Counsel to prove it.

Everyone had been asking me if I would get a divorce. I knew it was inevitable. I just wasn't in a rush because the Castle was in his dad's name. Not that they would throw me out. They knew as well as I did that J couldn't handle or run this business if his life depended on it. It would be messy. And he'd probably turn our house into a flop house like he did the SC. I had asked him earlier that day if he wanted a divorce. He said he never asked for one. I replied, "I asked if you WANTED one." Always competition.

I received a scathing, unsolicited by his own admission, letter from Ben:

Aloha Sheri,

I want to offer a little unsolicited advice, and I promise to do this only once. From the time you showed me around the castle a few months ago, I said, "You need to either fall in love with a handyman who wants to devote himself to this place, or you need to sell it."

This past weekend, I was a heartbeat away from having a fistfight with J at 4 a.m. while Leslie and I were in bed nude. I want to plead with you again to deal with reality and put the castle up for sale immediately so you can move on with your life before someone gets killed.

Sheri, the castle is a money pit that is never going to run smoothly or make a profit, and it needs more investment than you are capable of making. You and J have no mortgage. The lot itself could fetch a quarter million. You could probably have a quick sale of around $400,000, which would be split between you and J, and then you could GO YOUR SEPARATE WAYS AND NEVER HAVE TO DEAL WITH HIM AGAIN. You would have plenty of money to start a new life with.

Your friends, neighbors, and the local police have all been pulled into this horrible mess between you and J, and it is not going to get any better, no matter how many TROs you get. You need to STOP BEING INVOLVED IN HIS LIFE IN ANY WAY, and that cannot happen unless you sell the castle. You had a full house of paying guests Monday morning when the police showed up in two cars with blue lights flashing and told Leslie and me they could not arrest J because he did nothing wrong. He owns the place.

The TRO says nothing about him going inside or taking anything he wants. If I had punched him to protect my girlfriend, they said they would have arrested me for assault. We were in HIS HOUSE. From the police's point of view, if anyone was in the wrong, it was us. If Leslie agrees to help you in any way in the future, it will be the end of our relationship. It is three months between now and June. That is plenty of time to put the castle up for sale and make plans for what you are going to do for the next chapter of your life. I say all of this with love and friendship and concern for your well-being too. Please stop putting your friends in harm's way. Me ke aloha pumehana, Ben

Ben's words stung, though I knew he wasn't trying to be cruel. He was laying out the reality of the situation as he saw it—cold, clear, and final. Still, the weight of his ultimatum pressed down on me. The idea that my choices could cost me a friendship, that my actions had put people I cared about at risk, left a bitter taste in my mouth. Was I really being reckless, or was I just trying to hold on to something I wasn't ready to let go of? I wasn't sure.

I let out a slow breath and pushed those thoughts aside. There wasn't time to dwell. I was home, waiting for guests to arrive, after which I planned to try to sleep. I was determined not to smoke or drink. The 19th was my birthday and my target date to quit cigs again this year, like a New Year's resolution.

March 15

Yesterday, J called and asked if I had taken something from his flop house. I thought: me steal from him? Hey buddy, you stole from me, and I prescribed the don't stoop to his level mantra.

Today, he just called and wanted to know if we could talk and if I would cooperate to get some things accomplished. Me cooperate? How 'bout you first, Mister? He was so far from reality, it's remarkable. I told him that when he agreed that he would respect boundaries and my privacy, then we could talk. He started to say, "Well, it's clear …" I hung up.

March 16, 2012, Aunt Sheila's Birthday

I always call her to check in, wish her a happy day, and catch up. Miss her so much it's not funny. We had a nice chat and caught up.

March 17, 2012, St. Paddy's Day

I started taking anti-depressant drugs. I hate taking meds. Lorazepam and Citalopram. It had only been a couple of days, and I was trying to monitor myself. I woke up at 2 a.m. and then 4 a.m., but at least I was able to get back to sleep.

I met with the attorney, and he said he thought he could get the TRO done for $1,000, but he made no promises. Honestly, if I tried to handle it myself, I knew I'd lose. I was so depressed that I couldn't even imagine stringing together full sentences, let alone trying to argue my case in court. The thought of doing it alone was overwhelming.

I was supposed to meet him at court in Hilo on Monday at 8:10 a.m. and see if he could get it expedited by asking the clerk. If he pulled that one off, I swear I would have been in love.

J called wanting something—a phone number? My cooperation? What? I had no idea. Anyway, he told me that if I didn't give it to him or cooperate, things would not go well for me. Yet another threat. Did I really put up with this for twenty-two years? I was trying to remember what shield I had to protect me from his bullying. I told him that unless he agreed to what I wanted, we had nothing more to discuss. This is what I came up with:

WHAT DO I WANT? Besides peace and boundaries and some measure and assurance of security and privacy and safety? I want the following signed:

1. If you want or need anything from this property, call and request it, or if you feel you must come here, call to make an appointment.

2. Never set foot on the property without being invited or without me being here.

3. Never take anything from here, whether you think it's yours or mine or both of ours.

4. Never bring strangers onto this property. Especially in my bedroom or office EVER.

5. Bring back the propane tank you stole. I need it for the vacation rental business.

6. Pay for the van you stuck on my credit card—$2,000, register it in your name, and buy your own insurance.

7. Pay for your medical insurance $165/mo. It is 17 days late. I have been paying it since you left, and I'm done paying it.

8. Pay for half the credit card debt left at the time you vacated these premises on or about 12/1/11.

9. Joint custody of Bruiser. Either evenings or weekends. Preferably in a

block of time to minimize our contact with each other. I would request two to three nights per week.

If you cannot sign the above, what do you want? Can you state it without poetry or philosophizing?

I'm starving, but it is so hard to eat. I pulled out two eggs to fry early this morning and it's now 3 p.m., and I have yet to touch them. I'm down to 120 lbs.

March 18

OK, I must admit, I was a little scared. I just weighed myself: 118 pounds. I hadn't seen that weight since I was a teenager. Or on coke. I've got to get my hands on $800 for this attorney. I gave him $200, which covers going to court tomorrow, to try to get this date pushed up sooner.

So where were the sheriffs who were supposed to carry out the writ of possession on the spec house? I was hoping he would get himself arrested, and that would temporarily solve some of my anxiety by knowing he would be unable to come to the house and threaten me.

March 22

J called. Said he was coming to the house and that I should call the police. Then, as casually as if he were discussing the weather, he added: "If you don't give me what I want, I'll tear the house apart and kill you." Well, my mama didn't raise no dummy. I called the police and then two girlfriends to come and be with me.

When he arrived, he kneed me in the jaw, and scratched my girlfriend hard enough to draw blood, all the while screaming and spitting vile threats: "You are going to be sorry. I am the worst enemy you can ever have." He brought one of his homeless kids, who pulled his beat-up van into my driveway, leaking oil everywhere.

They left before the cops arrived, but couldn't drive since the van didn't start. They rolled it out into the park, where it now sits, so I could look forward to them returning to get it, I suppose. I called the attorney, who made it very clear I had to cough up more money.

March 23

Yesterday I learned that the judge granted the no-contact restraining order. A wave of emotions washed over me. Relief. Sadness, a flood of emotions, crashing over me all at once. It had come to this.

Later, Daniel, our architect, called to tell me that the job they had been waiting for would start soon, so J would have work. I prayed that the thought of a lucrative job would knock some sense into him and things might change, a turning point if you will.

I was glad I finally gave in to the meds—though God knows I resisted. But I had to admit, they were keeping me from hurling myself off the cliff. The only thing was that I'd have to take Ray with me. My gorgeous Rayba. My one constant. Those big brown eyes, always watching me. My soulmate.

March 25

I didn't know what I had done to make him hate me and want to destroy me. He had been threatening me almost daily and harassing me for his tools, his truck, and his phone. I don't even know why I bothered to write anymore. It felt pointless. I was so depressed I spent my days just waiting. Waiting for evening, waiting to take my pills, waiting until I could climb into bed with Ray. Waiting for the relief of sleep.

April 1

The no-contact TRO was in effect. My friend Cindy invited me for dinner, and I was trying to choke down some food when guess who strolled onto the property? Three guesses and the first two don't count. I told him, "You're not supposed to be here." He ignored me. He stayed and I left.

April 10

J called me, hysterical at 10:30 p.m. Bruiser had been attacked by a pit bull, and he begged me to come pick them up. Against my better judgment, I did. I know it was stupid. But I wasn't doing it for him, I was doing it for Bruiser. My anxiety surged so hard I was hyperventilating, to the point where I almost passed out. J demanded that I drive them to the vet immediately, which would have easily cost $500 for an after-hours visit. I refused and took them back to the SC. He was furious and said he would take him to the vet the next morning.

April 11

While running errands in Hilo, I stopped by the vet. Long story short? The bill was $100. J had left Bruiser there. He was waiting for me to pick up both Bruiser and the bill. What a guy!

April 13

I woke up to no electricity. Someone cut off the breaker and stole it. Someone. Gee, I wonder who. This was actually a blessing in disguise. A troubleshooter from Helco (Hawaiian Electric Light Company) came; he had the part and fixed it, and even helped me figure out a bunch of other electrical issues.

April 14

When I walked out to the driveway, both the Rav and the Echo had flat tires. CIH magnets on Rav gone. There was no water in the house. J changed all the valves to off, and the landline phone had been disconnected from the box. The dungeon door to the street was unlocked, so he came in through the deck and went out that door. The pool was off. What did he think? It would make me comply? Give back his phone, van, and tools. It was just the opposite. I wanted to go and sell all of it! Or burn it all in the street just for grins and giggles. I made a police report.

Then spent hours combing through surveillance footage, hoping to catch him on camera.

April 15

The phone rang. Olena Heu, a reporter from KHON2 was calling. She asked if she could come and do a piece on the Castle. Gulp. Of course. We decided on April 19, and I had to get hopping to get ready. The second I got off the phone with her, I started making preparations. The pool had to be cleaned, food for a spectacular dinner I wanted to cook for them had to be bought, as well as fresh flowers for their suites. I called my favorite massage therapist so I could gift Olena a massage before dinner. She was bringing her cameraperson so both suites would be utilized for their stay.

Ray needed a bath. I hated bathing him. Hated not bathing him. I had to bathe him. If I didn't, he got stinky. For the first time I thought maybe the "secret therapy" was helping a bit. Olena's visit wasn't hurting. I really did want and need professional help too. Talk therapy.

J called, rambling about 420. I'd never heard of it. Found out about it on wiki: cannabis culture slang for marijuana consumption, especially smoking around the time 4:20 p.m. It also referred to cannabis-oriented celebrations that take place annually on April 20. He said he was having a fundraiser at Uncle Roberts on 4/20 at 4:20 p.m. Is this what he wanted to be known for?

April 19

Olena and her cameraperson's stay was very successful. They did some b-roll (background). She got her massage before dinner as planned. I made them a Greek-style pizza on Naan bread, roasted veggies, and a huge rainbow salad, my kitchen sink salad as I called it. We had Haupia ice cream for dessert. Haupia is a traditional Hawaiian dessert made from coconut milk, and its flavor is rich, creamy, and mildly sweet. It was one of my favorites. I baked cookies as a gift for them to take.

Of course, right after they left, I thought about everything I had wanted to say during the taping but was too nervous and forgot to say. I received an email: "Sheri—thank you so much for a fabulous time! You are truly a gem, and we are so honored to know you! Mahalo nui loa, Olena." And their stay happened without any drama! Praise the Lord!

The piece would air in May for sweeps, and she would let me know as soon as she knew the date. During sweeps week, television networks aired their most highly anticipated shows, series finales, and specials to attract viewers and increase ratings. She said she would also send a DVD so I could post it on YouTube. I told J about the piece, and he had the balls to want to contact her, or wanted me to, to help him promote one of his causes. You know, the ones that didn't pay him anything. Shake head, roll eyes upward.

April 20

I was coming home from Pahoa at about 4:30, so I stopped at Uncle Roberts to get Bruiser. J was walking around. No one showed up for his 420 fundraiser. He was so delusional; it was sad. I took Bruiser and left.

April 21

I was just about to leave and go to town when J walked up and asked me to keep Bruiser because he had a meeting in Puna Palisades, a subdivision next to Seaview that was a couple of miles up the road. I wasn't planning on keeping the weenie, but I said OK.

I asked him if he wanted a ride. I didn't want to leave him at the house to get into trouble since the restraining order meant nothing to him. We barely made it a quarter mile before the drama started. We were discussing something that he didn't want to discuss. He declared, "Let me out!" The road was extremely narrow. There was no place to pull over, and I said, "Fine, let me get to a place where I can pull over." Before I could finish my sentence, he said, "I wish it didn't have to be like this." He flung himself out of the car at 30-35 miles an hour. Really? Was this something sane people do? What did he think would happen? His medical insurance had lapsed. I kept driving. Moments later an ambulance sped past me in the opposite direction toward where he'd jumped out of my car. He needed help. My girlfriend told me, "Don't feel sorry for him." I couldn't stop myself from feeling.

April 22

I was taking Ray and Bruiser out for a walk. We ran into a carpenter who had stayed at the flop house and left because of all the chaos. He told me it was the talk of Kehena Beach that I threw him out of the car. Raise eyebrows in disbelief. I was 120 pounds, he was 180 pounds. I was a peanut with little strength and not a violent bone in my body; he, on the other hand …I was driving a stick shift and could throw him out of the car? Then I got a message from a guy living at the flop house, who said, "You need to pick up prescriptions for J." Is that so? Dream on.

April 30

I was pulling out of my driveway to see my girlfriend, and two police cars passed by. There was only one road to my girlfriend's, so I had no choice but to follow to get to her house. I wondered what they were there for. When I got to my friend's house, J came out, and they stopped him! I thought, *Praise the Lord, it's over,* and I went into her house. About ten minutes later, they let him go and left the community. WHY did they do that? There were three APBs out for him.

May 1

I was going to take Ray for his final pee before nighty-night, and I heard whining outside the door, which I kept locked now. It was Bruiser. Fifteen minutes later, J yelled, "Give me my dog and my computer." I said, "I'll bring your dog, I don't have your computer." I threw on some clothes, grabbed the dog, and ran down the stairs, trying to figure out where he was. He was gone. I heard my car alarm going off. My neighbors screamed, "Sheri, are you all right?" I ran down the stairs and found an ax in my windshield and all the windows on the passenger side smashed, including the back windshield. I called the police. They came and watched the surveillance video, showing him leaving the property.

May 3

The auto glass guy came from Hilo and only had the front windshield for the Rav. He had to order the windows and said hopefully they would be there in a day. He asked me to go to his shop in Hilo so he could vacuum the car out better. Since I had to pick up guests at the airport, I decided to go prior to their arrival.

On the way to town, I stopped at Pahoa PD and got an audience with the captain. I let him have it—in my sweetest way, of course. Why did those officers not arrest him on Monday? He looked chagrined and said he'd check into it but couldn't tell me even if he did find out.

After ten years, I was used to the ineffectual ways of the system here. If they had done their job, I wouldn't be out a $250 deductible for the destroyed glass on my car. My girlfriend said there was a victim's fund, but there was no amount of money in the world that could compensate for the reign of terror I had lived through for the past six months.

I called my girlfriend Ellen to check in and check up on her. It turns out my intuition was at work. She had a loser ex-husband too. She said, "I just saw your husband at the gas station across from the police station."

My déjà vu nearly knocked me down. I told her to follow him while I called the police. The captain dispatched officers. J ran. They tased him. Dear Lord, please help this man while he is incarcerated. I'd tried to stay out of it. Let him dig his own grave. But this poor soul needed help. When I called the attorney to tell him what happened, he said, "I'm not surprised. I could see in his eyes that he was going to snap."

I organized an annual picnic for a thousand people in California for a loyal company I adored. As a thank you for their business, I gave them a free week at the castle to raffle. Ana won the complimentary stay, and I picked her and her partner up at the airport. On the way to get them, I wondered how I should explain why my car had no windows but ultimately decided to be honest and swore them to secrecy. They were the sweetest couple, and so grateful—it was their first vacation ever. OMG. We spent a great evening at Uncle Robert's. For the first time in six months, I finally felt like I could breathe.

May 8

While he was in jail, I enjoyed a few days of peace. I sank money into plumbers and a pool guy just to figure out how things worked. But once the bedroom door was fixed, I was pau (Hawaiian for finished or done).

It was low tide and a full moon. The well had no water. It was horrible to run around trying to find out why there was no water. At least I knew it wasn't the mischief-maker since he was in jail. And despite all the BS, I was still smoke-free. I must admit the accident almost pushed me to smoke, but I did not. Yippee. He would not win that. At 5 p.m., without fail, I still craved my nightly glass of red wine.

I needed a therapist to speak to. I forgot to call Bishop. He was supposed to get me help. Anyway, I wanted to try to remember feeling this calm. I didn't have to wear my keys and iPhone walking around my house in case I needed to take photos for evidence. I was not looking over my shoulder. Tomorrow was the day. Hmm. I wondered if he would get out.

His brother and his dad both called me. First, his brother screamed at me to give J his van and tools, then told me he would tell Dad to throw me out of the house if I didn't. Then Dad and his wife called and asked me what the hell was going on. I didn't know, but for some strange reason, I trusted them. Was I being stupid? Yes. That's why I needed a shrink. And an attorney. And money.

The latest drama was by a photographer who had me by the balls. I needed pictures for the CH, so I staged it, and she and her husband came over, spent an hour taking pictures, and told me I'd get the pictures in 48 hours. That was more than a week ago. We were doing it as a barter, but I guess she didn't want to do this, and they wanted cash. So instead of being honest, she made up some cock and bull story about how I was rude to her. Be rude to someone you want to do business with? I need a good photographer for weddings and such. In exchange for the barter, I told her I'd use her pictures on the website and give her credit, of course. She wrote me this:

"I will send the pictures to you when I have time. I am working on other clients and will not be rushed, especially on a favor! The way you have been treating us is not appropriate or professional. This service would cost anyone else upward of $5,000 or more. We specialize in high-end portraiture and weddings, and commercial photography does not do well in gaining clients for that medium; therefore, you stand to gain a lot more from this than us. The rude and demanding behavior is unacceptable and will not be tolerated."

She valued the hour they spent here at $5,000. Yikes. Most photographers in LA and Hollywood didn't gouge people that much. Cheri, my webmistress, wrote me: "My, my. Someone thinks very highly of themselves." I laughed and agreed.

May 9

I had to walk around the property constantly to see if the pumps were running and the pool was high enough. I was sick of it. Why couldn't this house just be normal and not hold me prisoner? I was happy my surveillance cameras were all working, but I couldn't wait to see if the company would trade me up. Their $100 cameras sucked and couldn't even seem to last two to three months in Hawaii.

I was still 118-120 lbs. and really loving it. However, I was also beating myself up because I wasn't doing something for my poor body. Who had time to exercise? And since Ray wasn't able to, I didn't care to. We were overrun with fire ants. It was terrifying. I cut some branches off a tree, and the f*ckers just dropped on me and bit me. And I couldn't even see them! That's when I decided to spend money and get Terminix to spray the property.

May 12

I am trying to monitor my mental health and depression levels now that I am off Chantix and cigarettes for four weeks. Maybe Chantix also helped with the depression, or else just being off the cigarettes lifted my mood and my spirits. My lungs felt so good!

I was really looking forward to Thalia coming over from Kona. She's a photographer I swear I manifested—she feels like my twin, my sista from anuda mudda. So sweet and thoughtful. She even wanted to clarify our deal in writing, which made me laugh. That's exactly something I would've said. She wanted to make sure she and her husband could come back another time after the shoot to actually relax, since he couldn't make it on this trip. It's funny, she must think I run this business like an actual business.

I was getting that CH whipped into shape, functional, and ready to rent. It took me two flipping hours to find two nails. I have at least 100,000 screws. As I organized, I kept finding crap I needed. Design of this house? Artistic, yeah. Functional? Not at all. I am fixing it to be both.

I couldn't help but feel envious of how dogs live so fully in the moment. I had to stop by the SC. Bruiser was with me in the car. Poor guy got so excited, thinking he was about to see his daddy. I told him, "No, Daddy's not here; he's in jail." In true dog fashion, he forgot about it moments later. I know I give him enough love, but he's really Daddy's boy, and I find myself overcompensating, feeding him all the good stuff. Today, he got a sheep fetus, and you should have seen how happy it made him. I had to cut it in half and smash the head so he could get to the brains. It was pure gold for him. Sad in a way, but once it's dead, it's just meat. Maybe I was a butcher in another life.

May 15

I'm driving on my way home from Kona. I had to go to Costco so I figured I'd take the dogs with me. Dog farts are HORRIBLE! I have all the windows open all the way. Whew. Ok, it's dissipating now. Tomorrow is court for J, and the DA called and said he would probably get out. Fabulous.

I knew Bruiser was looking forward to seeing him. Me? Not so much. Thalia was here Sunday and left Monday, and the pictures are unbelievable. I wonder how J is going to be when he gets out of jail. Remorseful or vindictive? This was a part of the "mental" I didn't understand. Thalia said it sounded a lot like bipolar.

I was all alone. What if I fell and couldn't get up? Sometimes, I loved being alone and getting things done uninterrupted. Other times, it was just plain lonely. Still smoke-free. For what? For who? Well, lungs are digging it.

May 22

I didn't go to church. I'm not comfortable leaving the house since J is out of jail. He told the court he was going to live at a friend's property in Ninoole, above Hilo. He lied. He went back to the SC. I don't know if he will come here and screw with something.

May 26

My crown on the front left side of my mouth came out. I snuck off to LA to get it fixed. Thank goodness the program with Hawaiian Airlines was so awesome. I could get back and forth to the mainland without going to the poor house! I had a feeling it wouldn't last. You got to fly unlimited for $2,500 a year. Too cheap, in my opinion.

In LA, I spent six hours in the dental chair on nitrous (yay), then went to stay with Maggie at her adorable little cottage in Marina Del Rey. It was a great, short trip. I also reconnected with a very dear old friend, Lou, who is an amazing man and a talented director and actor, and we went down memory lane. I've always been madly in love with him, not in a carnal way! With all the crap that I was going through, having a conversation with him was like coming home. He knew me from back in the 80s. We talked about Barry, and that was nice. I told him that Barry's next woman, after me, was also a Sheri Smith. He laughed and said what I thought, "What are the odds?"

Ray was famished. Poor baby, he only had about a pound of meat a day on this trip to LA. I took raw chicken in my luggage since time was at a premium, so I didn't have to shop. Usually, when I came back from LA, I took food home for myself. I would get something I couldn't get in Hawaii, usually Mongolian BBQ. I froze it, and it defrosted as I flew home. Then, I would have it for dinner.

I couldn't believe I had been nicotine-free for about six weeks. I found it hilarious that every other time I quit, I had a quit date. This time, I just did it and don't remember what date was the actual last day I smoked. It was supposed to be on my birthday, but I called it April 19, a month after. I was still craving one, but I didn't have one. Other quitters have said the craving never goes away.

The other exciting thing that happened in California was that Ray and I went to visit Cecilia. We had drama while we were there. Her dog, a pit bull, tried to hump Ray's head and dominate him. When Ray wouldn't have any of it, the dog attacked us. There was no blood, just a little pee. Me, not the dogs. We survived. If the dog had known what he was doing, we both would have been dead. I got Ray and myself into the bathroom on the floor in the dark and Cecilia got her dog outside the house. She kept screaming at me not to open the door. Was she

JOKING? My heart was pounding out of my chest, and I was hugging my boy in the dark on the bathroom floor. It was actually funny when I thought about it afterward, but at the time, I was terrified.

When I got back to Hawaii, J's new attorney served me with divorce papers, and he asked for support. What else is new? I had been carrying him for 22 years. He probably wanted me to support him for the rest of his life.

June 6

I'd always wanted to connect with someone I knew was going to the "other side." I'd been getting such psychic blasts of intuition and déjà vu lately and was trying to pay attention to them. I thought of Char, who had taught me so much, and I wanted to put her insights to good use. I was preparing a will and last directive so my wishes would be known and carried out. When I was married, I was pretty certain my wishes would never be respected. Horrible, isn't it? Now that I would soon be divorced, I'd made Brother

Jeff my executor, and I knew he would honor my last requests.

June 11

I am on my way to the mainland. I wanted to document today because it was a great and terrible day. I had a horrendous pain in my left hip. I thought it might be arthritis. I got to the airport, and for whatever reason, there was a problem with Ray's reservation for bulkhead, plus being in pain, they bumped me to first class. After I picked my jaw up off the ground, I was grateful for the blessing. I finally got the results of my X-rays. The doctor who saw me said I had a fractured back. It turns out it happened when I fell into the dungeon years ago.

August 18

I walked around the property checking valves, tanks, pumps, etc. I discovered the pipe for the hot tub was out of its housing. I called my neighbor to come and troubleshoot. When he got here, we went into the dungeon where the machinery for the jacuzzi was housed. A metal pipe was lying right next to the white PVC pipe that was out of place. There was a dent in the pipe as if it had been intentionally hit to damage the unit. I turned off the breaker; it was leaking pretty badly. Next, I needed to review the surveillance tape which would probably take me hours, with no guarantee that J walked past a camera.

September 21

Twelve years ago, when my husband wrote me a letter that said, "I'm sorry, I was wrong, it won't happen again, come to Hawaii, we'll heal," I took him at his word. I didn't get married to get divorced. Hell, I took him at his word a month or so ago when he told me, "I'll never divorce you," and five minutes later, he served me with divorce papers.

The judge had ordered him to let me have Bruiser one night a week. The last court date was two months before, and when he came to court on 9/1, he hadn't let me have him for all that time. At least I could have seen him for a few minutes in court, but he didn't bring him. How's that for hurtful?

Well, in a shocking turn of events, he dropped the dog at my girlfriend's house on Tuesday. She called me and said, "Bruiser's here, come and get him!" So yesterday, at about 6 p.m., I saw J in the park and reluctantly said my goodbyes to Bruiser. Then, with the magic words "Where's your daddy?" the little stinker started barking like crazy and raced out the door to find him. Bye, mama!

I had been praying nonstop. It's hard to be grateful when you're depressed, but I made it a point to count my blessings. I was in great health, and my dog had been going through some issues, but I thought we were past that now. I was doing quantum healing for him again. It had helped him two years earlier, though I wasn't sure if this time would be the same since his symptoms were different. I prayed we were finally over it. I had no visitors or guests and no catering. Things were looking bleak, but I focused on faith and knew God would take care of me in his time.

My attorney said we had to file a pleading (read: motion). What J's dad was doing was breaking a Constructive Trust, and he was enjoying unjust enrichment. I gave the attorney $3,000; he blew through all of it and wanted more. He had me by the balls. My hānai sister Mari, a brilliant patent attorney in Cali who loved challenges, ghost-wrote it, so to speak, and gave it to my attorney to "Hawaiian-ize" it to save me money.

If the house was sold, where would I go? What would I do? Cali was the only place I had a chance to make money. There were no opportunities in Hawaii, not for me anyway. I was too old to pick papayas. That depressed me too. I was an island child; I belonged in Hawaii. The blessing was I'd been able to live in paradise for the last ten years, so I would hang on to that.

September 23

That morning, I spent my time dealing with sheep. I had become a hunter and a butcher for my boy, getting animals at the base of Mauna Kea to be able to feed him raw. It was not really hunting. The rangers went up in helicopters, shot the animals, and dropped them to us so we could field dress them. Occasionally, a goat would be mixed in, and if I was lucky, someone would find a fetus. All the hunters knew I fed Ray raw, so if they found one, they'd call me over and give it to me.

I could barely eat. Nothing looked good, plus I didn't want to spend a penny. I went down to the propane tank. It seemed to be empty, and I thought it all leaked out. I had to be careful to turn it off after I used the dryer or cooked using the oven.

Besides the gas leak, the plumbing needed to be redone so I wouldn't run out of water every low tide. I lived in paradise and couldn't enjoy it. I wondered if everything worked, and if I had cash to function, then what? I'd still be alone and lonely.

I finally got visitation with Bruiser. When I brought him to the park to go back with J, I had to give him a bill, and he told me to put it in his van. There on the front seat was a big bag of pot. He was out there smoking with some guys, wearing his African beanie. Better than his Santa hat or Boy Scout shirt, I guess.

October 7

Someone gave me the idea to look for help on mindmyhouse.com. The website said:

"We provide all the online tools for home-owners and house/pet sitters to find each other from around the globe or around the corner since 2005." What a concept. Sorry, I didn't think of it! Sitters list why they want to sit and their qualifications. People contact you, and I would say 90% have experience, background checks, and references. Win-win. They come for various reasons and lengths of time. You give them a place to live, and they take care of your place while you're away. The only thing is trying to keep all the applicants/candidates straight. It was a lot.

Maggie said if she produced a show on HGTV, I could work as PA or perhaps do craft services. Things weren't certain yet, and she would keep me in the loop. Darkest before the dawn, right?

Hawaii is an equitable distribution state. Meaning that if the parties in a divorce can't agree, the property will be distributed equitably, not necessarily equally. Mari suggested I pursue this course of action. In making these orders, the court would take into consideration the respective merits of the parties, the relative abilities of the parties, the condition in which the divorce will leave each party, the burdens imposed upon either party, and all other circumstances of the case.

If the case was presented properly, I could (and should) ask for the house and furnishings. The other thing was my attorney. I struggled to decide whether he was indeed a "good" attorney and the "correct" one. I had a sense that he was not.

October 9

Another day, another no dollar. What was going on? There weren't even any inquiries, and even if there were, I couldn't book them the way the house was. Food stamps next? Another first. A new low. It was a hot, sunny day, but instead of enjoying it, all I had to look forward to were attorneys and court. What fun! I've been trying to sell stuff on Craigslist and eBay, but it's a slow, tedious process—especially when you're technically challenged like me.

Sunday, my bathroom jacuzzi tub on the third floor caught on fire. Huh? How? Why? I was hysterical. What else could possibly go wrong? As I sat there, I realized what depressed me most was the thought of starting over at 58. Even if the judge awards me the house, then what? I'd never feel safe as long as J stayed in Seaview, not after all the violence he committed.

If I could choose, I'd love to work as a personal assistant to a celebrity chef. Alex Guarnaschelli? Cat Cora? Definitely no men—especially not the one who cheated on his wife with my friend. I was disillusioned with men.

October 18

Last night, a group of us went to Uncle Robert's to "talk story" (Hawaiian expression for chat or shooting the breeze). It was a lovely time, until guess who showed up? J was supposed to leave if we were in the same place and the other was already there. As usual, he didn't. He never did. So, I left. Thankfully, we'd been there a while and had already finished eating, so at least it didn't ruin my night completely.

I've taken to talking to myself. It could be misconstrued that I was talking to my boy. It started as early as 4 or 5 a.m. I opened my eyes and those gorgeous big brown eyes were staring into mine. I tried to shake out the cobwebs and beg him for a bit of space, but no, he didn't give an inch. If I wasn't fast enough, in his opinion, to respond to his conversation, which was all non-verbal, he would then move from his crouching position, chin on the bed, and come and sit on me. Then he would look away. His next step in this dance: he mouthed off and barked until I gave in. I say, oooooooo-K. After that, he was pretty amenable in terms of letting me make coffee before we went out, but I think he knew that it was not negotiable. Mama needs coffee when she wakes up.

I gave him his thyroid pill before we headed out, and sometimes, as the coffee brewed, I would check my email on Lucious, my nickname for my iPhone. Now that I was alone, I walked around naked. How freeing! No titillation here, just nature at its best. Dog naked, mama naked. He didn't judge me for my wrinkles, my weight or my flab. No matter what I weighed, I always saw flab.

I quit quitting cigs yet again. I had made it to six months but started again. If I had a pack, I smoked a pack; if I had two, three, or four cigs, that's how many I smoked. There was a convenience store at the end of the road that sold single cigarettes—totally illegal, of course. Another option was getting them in plastic baggies, hand-rolled by someone with a machine, complete with filters. Also illegal, definitely a market for it, considering how expensive the "real" ones were in Hawaii.

I finally got a mental health crisis manager! I get to see him once a week—thank the Lord. I've been grappling with the possibility of having to move back to California, which would absolutely break my heart. The reality is, I can't afford to live in Hawaii on my income alone. There was no fork in my road coming up; it was an octopus of avenues. And to make matters worse, a stranger—a judge—would decide my fate and future on January 11. I was trying to stay open to all possibilities, but the uncertainty weighed heavily on me.

2013

January 15

My mental health crisis manager had just left, and I felt a bit better. Fighting depression was a full-time profession, I must say. I got Marianne Williamson's book *A Return to Love,* and, in a nutshell, I was trying to choose love. The other option was choosing fear. I had to keep repeating this to myself. And keep remembering that nothing good ever came from being fearful.

I got a FB message from "Char's staff," saying she was looking for people to share their intuition experience. I posted:

> The experience that I want to share involved Char. In the '90s, Char came to California to shoot her video "Questions from Earth, Answers from Heaven," and my company, Gourmet Catering, had the honor and privilege of catering it. I was already a big fan, so I wanted to be there.
>
> As I was leaving my house, I felt I should bring vitamins, particularly vitamin C. When I got there, I asked her if she was feeling well, and she said she thought she was getting a little cold, so I whipped out the vitamins to help her combat the bug.
>
> Soon after that, I got a personal reading, and she told me the name of my dead dad, Nat. She also gave me a signed copy of her book and took a picture with me, which I have hanging on the wall of my office.

Connecting with Char was the most profound experience of my life and one I will always be grateful for. Much aloha and blessings. My castle has a suite with your name on it, should you ever feel you'd like to come to paradise to recharge.

They posted it and wrote: Thank you so much for sharing your story!

HOME STRANGE HOME on HGTV contacted me. The producer said they wanted to plan to come Feb. 6, 7, and 8. I wasn't holding my breath until I got the "it's finalized" call or email.

Update on the castle status. I got caretakers from the MindMyHouse website. Ron and his wife Jade and Ron's brother Alex had done an amazing job bringing this castle to its knees. That's not to say there wasn't a ton of crap to do and money to spend to make it "all" right, but they made it so that it's tolerable to live here, not living in fear that something is leaking or needs fixing or cleaning. And this place sparkled. Ron tended to talk story (as they say on the island) a lot. He went off on tangents. Hey, he was me. J used to call me Edith Bunker. Jade spent most of her time chained to her computer. She was me too! We all had issues with alcohol. The boys and I had issues with nicotine. They didn't want to quit; they just talked about wanting to.

Jade was supposed to go back to the mainland. Hopefully, she would go alone. Ron and Alex wanted to stay, which would be a good thing. Ron wanted to live on the Big Island; she wanted to go home to Utah in the summer and enjoy the mountains.

This has been a truly remarkable experience. I asked to manifest a nuclear family, and boom. They had been here since mid-September, and it had mostly been a positive learning experience. All families, whether blood, foster, or modern, have issues. It's how much you want to work them out. I wanted to work them out, and I think Ron did too. It was just the alcohol that I was fearful of. When Jade drank, she screamed at me. However, having said that, we were all great at going to our separate spaces, processing, cooling down, or sleeping it off and coming back together with acknowledgment and apology, if necessary, and then going on with our life in paradise.

I had gone from wanting to walk away—no, run away—to doing an about-face, determined to follow through with the plans, to focus and finish. All that stood in my way was a boatload of money. My next hare-brained idea—or as J would have said, "And for your next act?"—was to go on **Shark Tank**. The show was becoming a huge phenomenon, and it completely captured my imagination. OK, maybe I was a little obsessed. There was just one small problem—I didn't have a product to sell.

I had decided that I would draw out this divorce for as long as possible until I got my f*cking house into my f*cking name. How did I really feel? Can you hate someone and still forgive them? That's what kept rattling around in my head. Can you forgive someone and still hate them? I think so. Because I had to forgive him. He was sick.

My dear friend Maggie was going through some rough times, and I tried to reach out to her, but I knew what her schedule was like. I was chained to my desk and computer most of the time but had the luxury of stopping and connecting. She was having an affair with a married guy, and he was treating her like crap. Textbook. Been there, done that. He knew about me! Well, he knew about the castle anyway. Maggie texted him while they were on break. She promised to get to Hawaii and come visit in September. Fingers, toes, and eyes crossed.

Laura, bless her, has been my rock. She not only lent me money, but she also gave me personal and moral support—just as important, if not more so. Just hearing her voice had a way of calming me. Panic attacks are no joke, but Laura was always there, even from the East Coast. In some ways, it was a blessing since she was five (sometimes six) hours ahead of Hawaii time, so she was always available when I needed her most. She tried to teach me how to be alone, and for her, it was effortless. She never felt lonely. I, on the other hand, was struggling with loneliness.

Ray had been having issues again, and every time it happened, it sent me into a tailspin. I couldn't focus or concentrate. All I could do was worry. Meanwhile, Brother Jeff was caregiving his girlfriend. I felt bad for him because he never got to experience life with someone healthy like he was.

My neighbor up the road, "Old" Kelly, was coming to shower. Ron and Alex told me they would try to help him fix his water situation. His house was a ramshackle. His partner had passed away, and he lived on social security which was minimal. I tried to help him in whatever way I could.

January 21

At 9 p.m., someone threw fireworks at the gate. It wasn't just a little burst, it was a full-on barrage. It went on for a solid five minutes, loud enough to rattle the windows. It scorched the grass in front of the rock wall. I saw it from my bedroom window on the third floor. My heart pounded as I went to investigate, Alex close behind. As I walked past the CH, I glanced in and saw Ron passed out in the chair—probably drunk if he didn't hear the ruckus from the fireworks. Yesterday, it was Jade passed out in the same spot, all day. Their alcoholism was distressing.

They were supposed to be renting the Echo for $500 a month, but on Saturday, they came back home with a '94 SUV. So now the money I'd been counting on from the Echo's rental, which I planned to use for taxes, was gone. Jade called me a liar. She claimed I told them I'd sell the Echo for $2,500, but I never offered the car for that price. I've never lied to them about anything. I was furious. I had the car listed for $3,200 and had three serious buyers lined up, but I let them go so Jade and Ron could rent the car while living at the castle.

Another time, we were playing the card game *Weed*. Jade was probably lit, as usual. She tended to get emotional and blow up over anything and everything after a few drinks. She again accused me of lying. I decided then I wouldn't play cards with her after that. In fact, I didn't want to be around her at all when she was drinking.

Yesterday, I took Ray to the vet in Hilo and got him a shot of Adequan. I'd missed Dr. J's calls for two days, and I was desperate to consult with him about this. I was willing to try anything to help my boy. It was expensive, but if it worked, it would be worth every penny. This felt like my last ray of hope—pun intended. I couldn't even begin to imagine life without him. Watching him in pain was unbearable. I kept promising him, "Mama will get you better, Mama will fix you." Please, God, don't make me a liar.

I fought depression daily. I was back on the "aunties"—my name for the anti-depression and anti-anxiety pills. And I started smoking again. I had been taking walks around the park since Ray's stamina was shot. It was my way of pretending to exercise, while he could just lie in the middle of the park, keeping an eye on me as I looped around. I even dragged myself to a couple of yoga classes, though I've never really liked yoga. I slipped back into being a slug. My desk was piled high with things I needed to do—taxes, checklists, and proposals for picnics—and yet, I was constantly exhausted, barely able to keep my eyes open, falling over tired.

January 25

I went to bed at 10 and woke up at midnight. I took some tart cherry, hoping it would help me get back to sleep. I guess I did after an hour. At 3 a.m. Ray came to the bed and started whining. I was still trying to learn his "I gotta go" whine from his "I'm in pain whine."

I started down the stairs, and he bound after me, so I figured it was "I gotta go." We went down the stairs, and he practically ran to the grass and peed and pooped. It was so unusual for him to go in the middle of the night. Since we came back at 5 p.m. from a long ride to Kona and back, I guessed I didn't give him his last potty break late enough. I was gripped with fear in the pit of my stomach when he had episodes. Since stairs aggravate his condition, it was horrible to have to have him go up and down to relieve himself.

At 6 a.m., same thing. He ran out urgently, peed long and hard, then pooped. At 11:30 a.m., he peed long but drippy. It looked like his tummy might be bloated. I left word for Dr. J. I was not sure if I was getting hysterical or if I should take him to the vet in Hilo. He was supposed to go anyway for another injection of Adequan, but I was not sure if I should be adding this into his "mix" or not. It was so difficult to know the right thing to do. I couldn't work; I couldn't concentrate; all I could do was worry.

January 26, Larry's birthday

I called Larry as soon as I woke up to wish him a happy birthday since it was six hours later for him on the East Coast. We chatted for a bit, then I took off to the farmer's market in Hilo. I wanted to make a gorgeous superfood salad when I got home (kale, Brussels sprouts, spinach, broccoli), and whatever else I found at the market. Meanwhile, here I sat, puffing on a cigarette. I will say, in my defense, that I was also trying to figure out the e-cig solution. I was researching the best one for the best price, made in the USA. I wanted one where I could control the nicotine level, so I researched as I sat puffing and drinking a can of poison—Mountain Dew—my favorite caffeine delivery system.

Lately, my morning routine has been dealing with Ray's food, getting all my vitamins together, and taking the aunties. I didn't feel they were working, but I knew they needed time to build up in my system.

Yesterday, J was riding his bike around the park, not in front of the house, but on the other side, and I still felt him, so I looked out the window and saw the African beanie. I walked into the park, whistled for Bruiser, and he came running. I got a few minutes of love. He missed his mama as much as his mama missed him.

The producer of *Home Strange Home* emailed:

Sent: Monday, January 28, 2013, 7:44 a.m.

To: Sheri Smith

Subject: Still up in the air

Hi Sheri,

The Executive Producer decided against a Hawaii special in the end, but we are still going to pitch your home, along with a few others, for *Home, Strange Home,* and hopefully we'll get to shoot them still. I will keep you posted. I already have your casting sheet ready to go and will let you know when I have more information.

Ruth had taken to calling to harangadoodle me to try to extract the money we owed her. Her husband called me, drunk, in the middle of the night to do the same. They were still separated; I think he was on the West Coast, and she was in New Jersey. I felt bad but tried to make it very clear that I would honor my commitment when I was able.

April 2013

The alcoholic trio finally left, replaced by a new couple—Sheila and Carter. They seemed nice enough, and I was excited to learn she was a chef, which I loved! I wasn't so sure about him, though—time would tell. We sat on the moat deck, sipping wine and enjoying the view as J circled the park between 7 and 7:45 p.m. We watched in total amazement. He was supposed to pass the house only to enter and leave the community, not every ten minutes. There were so many more violations that I lost count. The justice system and police in Hawaii were so inept, inefficient, and ineffective that it became laughable.

When we woke up, I took the dogs to the park and noticed something brown. I thought it was the mango tree shedding dead bark or something. Sheila said it didn't look like it came from the tree; it looked like something was burned. I said, "Hmmm, I guess we should look at the video."

We looked and the time and date stamp said 11:23 p.m. J came onto the property on his bike. He wandered around on the ground floor, entered the Breezeway kitchen, and then into both suites. I didn't have them locked. Then, on his way out, he set something on fire. I think it was a rag or something; I wasn't sure if he was trying to blow up the Echo since he did it right behind the car.

We called the police. An officer came, we watched the video, and he said it was too dark and grainy to make a positive ID. Sheila and I were incredulous. How could he not recognize that scraggly Santa beard down to his waist? The most unbelievable part was that he did it while Bruiser was visiting. If Bruiser had done his job and alerted us, we all would've woken up, and we might have caught him in the act. I later contacted the sergeant in Pahoa, hoping they could enhance the video. No luck. Apparently, I've been watching way too much *Law and Order*.

April 19

I was walking Ray around 8 p.m. when I saw a crowd of people gathered in the park in the dark. A pickup truck had its headlights on, and there was J, dancing around in the middle of it all. I thought it was odd but didn't think much more of it. We went home.

April 20

At about 1 a.m., I jolted awake. No idea why. I stepped outside and walked into the park. Sure enough, there was J's pickup. I called the police, and at about 3 a.m., they finally came, but he was gone. A man and a woman were sleeping in his truck. The cops left, and so did I.

I went out again around 6 a.m., just after sunrise, and started taking pictures. I called the police and they arrived at 7 a.m. After measuring the distance to the house, they confirmed that he was in violation of the protective order—yet again. I urged the officer to check at the SC for him, and they headed up the community to investigate.

The woman and man in the car told me they lived at Cinderland, an intentional community a few miles down the road. It had crude shelters for sleeping, a kitchen, restrooms, etc. I offered them coffee and a ride home. On the way, the woman started filling my ear. She told me J was on LSD the previous night. He told them he fancied himself as Robin Hood. He was using someone's Home Depot credit card, taking from the rich and giving to the poor (himself).

As we drove down the red road, who do you think we saw jogging toward us—looking like he was wearing a diaper? I immediately flipped a U-turn and sped back to the SC. Thankfully, the officer was still there. I told him we'd just seen J up the road. The officer took off in that direction, and we pulled over to give him enough time to catch up and hopefully make the arrest.

When I got back from Cinderland, about 20 minutes later, I was confused to see J back at the truck in front of the castle, spray-painting it orange. I thought they would have arrested him earlier. Suddenly, three police cars appeared, and they arrested him. Hala-freaking-luya. Bruiser was with him, so I asked the cops if I could have Bruiser. They said yes. I went back to the house with him to celebrate.

An hour later, I went to the park to move the car so the neighbors wouldn't see it and gossip. The battery was dead, and there was no gas. A transient hippie with long hair and beard, sunglasses, tattered clothes, flip-flops, and a backpack was walking away from it. I imagine he took stuff, as I didn't see J's laptop or phone. Who knows, who cares?

I grabbed a gas can which had a gallon in it, jumped his truck with my car, and drove it up the main drag of the community, parked it in front of the SC. As I got out, I noticed his wallet on the floor in the back. There was a Home Depot card and a huge wad of receipts. After I got home, the sergeant called to tell me they'd taken him to the hospital for a tox screen. Please, God, I hope so! Bail was set at $4,000.

I dropped the receipts off to the police on my next trip to Pahoa.

Who said, "Most people lead lives of quiet desperation"? I swear I'd been feeling a lot of that lately. Quiet desperation. Don't get me wrong, I was a big believer in *The Secret* and *The Law of Attraction*, but lately, quiet desperation had been describing me.

I couldn't imagine living in California, New York, or Las Vegas anymore. The first time I set foot on a Hawaiian Island, it was Maui. I was in my late twenties, and I knew I was an island child. I was home. That was it. I knew one day I would live in Hawaii. Now, seeing the names and dates on the headstones in our pet cemetery in the yard, I can't bear the thought of leaving them behind if I had to leave. The cats: Punkin, Bu Kitty (Malibu), Gwen, Merlin. The dogs: Molly and Sam. They've all been a part of my life.

November 11

At about 2 in the morning, a car pulled into my driveway. I went out to see who it was or what they wanted and was shot in the arm with a BB gun. I called the police, made a report, but as usual, nothing was done.

KSECA (Kalapana Seaview Estates Community Association) Board of Directors appointed me as the Safety Committee chair due to the violence and vandalism that has recently escalated in our community parks. I wrote this letter to the Board:

Beatdowns, black eyes, assault and battery. Tagging of mailboxes and tampering with mailbox locks, which I believe are federal offenses. Vandalism of our bulletin boards, tearing up the grass with vehicles doing donuts, and spewing cans of paint everywhere. It sounds like LA but it's here in Seaview. I found fires on the grass in the front park along with dirty diapers, and feces. One night, a car pulled into my driveway and I was shot with a BB gun. I contacted the police about these matters and asked for our community officer to attend this meeting … but apparently, he is not here.

Having had the privilege of dealing with the PD and the court, unless you had video and photos, people would not be brought to task for their crimes. It was as simple as that. They do it because they know they can get away with it. Because we're so remote, the cops never show up when crime happens. The first thing the cops ask: is there video? I am asking for funding and a budget for the tools that would help us be safe and to identify and catch these criminals. Namely to have video surveillance. We all deserve some expectation of safety in our own backyard. When you go anywhere, such as Walmart or Target, you know you are being taped.

The community's rock wall was broken at a cost of some $3,000. If that money had gone to surveillance, we wouldn't even be having this conversation. We should be able to maintain safety in our parks and use them safely. As a deterrent to what I have described, I ask and make a motion that we buy video surveillance cameras and a system, including but not limited to night vision, low or no light, and the budget to pay for labor to install it immediately by our new board to accommodate our three parks for our protection and prevention of future crime.

It didn't happen.

2014

January 12

Paraliminals were a true blessing in my life, a lifeline actually. The website claimed they could "improve any aspect of your life in just 20 minutes a day—even while you're sleeping!" Energy in 10 minutes, memory boost in 16, mood lift in 18, new habits in 24. It sounded like exactly what the doctor ordered, so I gave them a try. Later I would credit them with saving my life.

March

At NPE, Ray was declining faster and faster, and it was time for him to go, but I couldn't let him go. I'll never forget being in the valet parking of the Hilton. He had diarrhea all over the place. I felt horrible for those poor kids who worked valet. I called Dr. J, and he graciously said, "Bring him to me." I took him to his veterinary hospital in Santa Ana, and Dr. J cleaned him up and took care of him so I could finish attending the convention. He is such a dear friend and kind person. I love him so much.

April 8, 1:32 p.m.

I killed my boy. People tell me, "Don't say that—say euthanized, put down." Seriously? How about destroyed? Dead is dead. I did my duty. I killed him because his quality of life sucked. I probably waited two weeks too long to do it. It feels just like the debate between Dementia and Alzheimer's—who cares what you call it? They both suck.

I know dogs don't last that long, but to lose my boy at only seven years is ridiculous. My heart dog, my baby, my soulmate. It is said when you lose an animal, you gain an organ that secretes sadness for the rest of your life. Yes indeed. Felt like the sun and the moon vanished.

Watching the needle go into his arm and take his precious life was just too much to bear. I wrote a script about it and him, called PeopleMakePlans.com. Most people would write a book, a novel, a blog. Not me. I was not like most people. Something in me was trying to get out after Ray's death and the emptiness that consumed me. I had to write, or I would expire. I'd written screenplays before so that part was easy. I had no clue how to write a book. The only thing I couldn't do at first was to make the script the proper length. As it poured out of me, it grew to 120 pages. The best page length in the industry is 90 pages. A page translates to one minute; a feature film is typically 90 minutes. I wasn't thinking about that. All I was thinking about was grief that had to come out.

On June 27, Kīlauea reminded us who's boss. Lava from the Puʻ uʻ Ōʻ ō vent was creeping towards Pāhoa like some kind of slow-motion nightmare. There I was, finally free from cigarettes, only to have Mother Nature force-feed me smoke and ash. On November 10, 2014, it reached and damaged the Pahoa Recycling and Transfer Station. The facility, valued at around $3.9 million, probably sustained about a million dollars in damage. It also claimed my girlfriend's house in the area nearby.

The lava threatened to cut us off from the rest of the island. We were a community of approximately 1,000, and would be left without supplies! How could I keep taking bookings and money when I couldn't guarantee people would even be able to reach the castle? My gut told me it was time to go. Time to say goodbye to the dream and face reality. The Big Island didn't feel so big anymore, and my little corner of paradise had turned into a danger zone. Sometimes, you've got to know when to fold 'em. Right

Kenny Rogers? By November 15, 2014, I was on a plane back to the mainland.

Life came full circle. I wasn't naive—I knew J would move into the castle the second I left. I just had no idea just how bad things would get. Pedophiles, meth heads, a whole parade of low-lifes. He turned our home into a haven for the worst of mankind. It stopped being a home the second I left; it became a house of horrors when he moved in. Little did I know he'd invite such unsavory humans into what was once our sanctuary. I headed back to Fullerton, the place I had come from. I packed everything that I'd spent a nickel on.

I packed what I could into a 20-foot container. The ward members were incredibly kind, helping me box everything up. Once I got back to Southern California, I rented a storage space in Fullerton and put everything there until I could figure out my next move.

I reached out to FDS, who had been with Gourmet since the 90s. Over the years, he became more than just a colleague—he was a dear friend, my "work husband," as I fondly called him. Coming from a large family of thirteen siblings—two of whom had passed away young—many of his family members also worked for Gourmet. I'll never forget one December, during our peak season, his father even came from Mexico to lend a hand. FDS's generosity didn't stop there. Whenever I traveled back and forth from Hawaii, he would graciously give up his bedroom for Ray and me, ensuring we always felt at home. His kindness and unwavering support meant the world to me, especially during moments when I needed a true friend by my side.

I chose Long Beach to try to find a rental house. Since I lived in Long Beach, Long Island, back in the '70s, I figured how could that be wrong? It was in between Fullerton near FDS and Los Angeles near PP. The neighborhood was the pits, but I found a clean three-bedroom, two-bathroom house that I could afford with a roommate. I found the roommate, but he turned out to be another bully, and Brother Jeff helped me get rid of him.

I landed back where I started as if I had been abducted by aliens and plopped back down with nothing when they were finished with me fifteen years later. I headed for the Mormon church in Fullerton for fellowship, knowing I'd be welcomed with open arms by people whose warmth and acceptance are simply a reflection of who they are.

Coming from a place where it rained constantly back to this place with its drought was very traumatizing. From constant rain to drought—it felt unnatural. If you watched me brush my teeth, you'd laugh. Wasting a drop of water felt criminal.

When I first got back, I knew I needed an animal in my life. A dog was out of the question—I just couldn't handle it. The loss of Ray was too raw. Instead, I volunteered at German Shepherd Rescue of Orange County (GSROC) for some much-needed puppy love. I've loved the breed since I was a child, but I knew I could never own another GSD. While I was there, one of the kennel workers mentioned that their cat had a litter of three kittens. I took them all, knowing I'd keep one and find homes for the others. That's exactly what happened. Two were black, and one was black and white. I named the male black kitten Black Magic, hoping he'd work some on my heart.

One day, while driving down the street, I pulled up next to a police car at a red light and flashed him the heart sign. He looked confused at first, so I made it obvious. I touched my heart and extended my hand. He caught on and said, "Thank you for your support." I told him, "I can't even imagine how you do what you do." He smirked, "I go to therapy and drink alcohol". I cracked up. Nice that he has a sense of humor. He looked like he was about 30, so I jokingly added, "Too bad you're way too old for me."

At the next red light, I looked at the car to my left and saw my balloon artist from the '90s who used to work for GC! His name was Bill. His clown name was Gumdrops, I called him Gummy. What were the chances? We exchanged phone numbers before the red light turned green.

In the next few months, we got reacquainted and spent time together and it was just like old times, which was heartening. He was always so kind and generous. Joanne, his wife, and I got to know each other better since we hadn't spent too much time socializing back in the day when Gummy worked for Gourmet. We became dear friends. I called her JoJo. She hated that. She was a caregiver to her granddaughter, who had cerebral palsy and then to her husband when his health started to decline.

I reconnected with one of my team members. His mama had Alzheimer's, and she couldn't utter one intelligible sentence. It was so sad. He changed her diapers and fed her; he did whatever it took, and my heart went out to him. He put his life on hold to be her caregiver. He's a hero in my mind.

My cousin got in touch with me. I was not sure how he found out I was back on the mainland.

He called me, and I told him, in no uncertain terms, that I was not interested in drama at this time. He was an expert at that. I only wanted to connect with my Mom and her husband, catch up, and see how they were doing. I missed her and didn't know her husband well or personally. I wanted to spend time with them and get to know him.

For some reason, I was suddenly obsessed with getting into shape. More than that, I needed community. I shopped three gyms, and Gold's Gym won. I did the machines and watched all the unique and different bodies as they passed. Trying not to make judgements. Big butts, little butts, no butts, my butt. I swam 30-60 minutes a day. It was the least I could do for myself, I figured. I felt like a bubbling volcano, ready to spew any minute—an ironic metaphor since I had just been house-cleaned by Madame Pele, which is how the natives refer to the lava. When the lava started to flow, we called it Pele cleaning house. The people who weren't supposed to be on the Big Island, who couldn't handle it, would leave. At that time, I knew I would be one of those.

I wanted to write and help anyone who might have lived through a similar situation. Similar? I silently laughed right after the word hit the page. Reality check. I had to eat and pay rent. All I knew how to do and could do well was to be an event coordinator or event specialist. I was determined never to have a kitchen again. I preferred putting an event together on paper. I didn't need a kitchen; I had too many friends who already had a kitchen, a team, and/or a chef. At one time, they were competitors, but if you conducted your business with integrity, you could call them friends. That was one of the important lessons PP taught me, among many others.

One of these people was Frank. I reached out to him, and we got together. He was happy for me to sell, and he would execute my events. After about a year, his wife decided we couldn't be friends. Scratch head here. I guess she was jealous of me, and I had no idea why. He and

I had no romantic inclinations; it was just the opposite. He was my caterer for nonprofits and organizations that didn't have huge budgets. So we stopped speaking and texting and being friends. It was awful for me, but if he had a happy marriage, so be it.

The other person was my dear friend Henry, who had a 5,000-square-foot kitchen. He was a chef who grilled a mean tri-tip! And tri-tip is on most of the menus I sell for picnics. I would put together a proposal for an event, and he would tell me what he would charge for the food and kitchen labor. I was fine with that. I was happy to coordinate and do the entertainment, rentals, and whatever else was needed for the event. I wanted no part of kitchen ops.

Another person I reconnected with was Lynette, J's first ex-wife. When I booked events, I would always staff (hire) her first. While we have different personalities, she knew as much as I do about running events, having done it as long as I did in the beginning with J. And we became dear friends. She is a good person. I'm so glad she said she would be on my team! Then, she moved to Utah to be closer to family. That sucked.

I'm determined to have a relationship with my Mom even though I haven't seen her in the fifteen years I lived in Hawaii. I always called her and kept in touch to find out what she was up to and tell her what was happening in my life. She and Don never came to see the house I built. I kept begging them to visit, but they were always too busy with golf and traveling—some things never change. It didn't matter much since we always stayed in touch by phone. Still, I wished we had written letters to each other like we used to. I had kept every single one she ever wrote me. After getting settled, I called and made plans to drive to Vegas. I was both anxious and excited to see her after all those years. I missed my Mommy!

Magic and I hit the road for Vegas, his litter box in tow, for a week-long visit with Mom. Watching her bond with Magic melted my heart and brought back memories. I couldn't help but recall the summer I returned from camp with Shadow, also a black cat who she allowed me to keep. Over time, she grew fond of Shadow, just as she did with all my pets.

While I was there, I cooked for her and Don. I loved how she called him Donald when she wanted to emphasize something, as a mom does with a child. It was good to be home. I felt a sense of relief. The past was forgotten, and bygones were bygones. I got to know Don, who I'd never spent time with up until this point.

Mom dedicated countless hours tending to his website, pouring her heart into preserving his legacy. She often sought my advice, knowing I had previously designed GourmetCatering.com and the CastleInHawaii website. I was honored to be part of her mission. It meant so much to her to keep his legacy alive.

2015

This year was all about piecing my life back together in California. With my restraining order in place, I was enrolled in VINE (Victim Information and Notification Everyday). Every time he went in or out of jail, VINE called and notified me. Apparently, he got into a fight at the SC and punched someone. He was sentenced to ten years but was released after three years and placed on parole. He was diagnosed with bipolar disorder, though I doubt he took his medication.

He was sent back to jail. Oh well, it's not my problem anymore.

I had signed up for Hawaii PD text alerts. I could have canceled them, but emotionally, I just couldn't. I thought that if anything happened at the castle, at least I'd be the first to know. I longed for my castle, but I lost the castle. I needed to: "Let go, let God", as the saying goes. Lesson learned: A constructive trust must be in writing. Signed. Even with family.

Determined to share my boy's story, I started marketing the script, hoping for a development deal. I joined a website that connects writers with producers, where you can pitch your logline, synopsis, and a personal message. I also entered contests to see if the script was any good. It earned a few honorable mentions but never first prize.

During this time, I pitched to and later met Jeff—a producer, writer, and director. He said his genre was horror, but he read the script and told me he would try and help. Long story short, we became friends. To distinguish him from

Brother Jeff, I called him Producer Jeff. I joined LinkedIn and started making connections, hoping to find other producers to pitch to.

I'd been wanting to plan a trip to New York City to spend time with Aunt Sheila and finally made it happen in October 2016. We had a wonderful time together, picking up bialys for me to take home—something I could never find in California. We visited a pickle shop with my girlfriend Heidi. We went to my all-time favorite restaurant, Serendipity, famous for its nostalgic atmosphere and incredible desserts. Laura, Larry, Fran, and their son Eric and his toddler —all of whom lived outside of the city—made the trip to join us, making it an even more memorable gathering.

2016

Poor Aunt Sheila. Last year, she was fine. This year, her memory was gone. She asked me four times, every five to six minutes, "Have you spoken to your mother?" I answered, and she asked me again. I wanted to cry. I don't want to get Alzheimer's or dementia or whatever she has. I want someone to shoot me if that happens.

Don Cherry, Mom's husband, was a singer and celebrity golfer. I found his wiki with all his accomplishments and the albums he made.

He was a good man; he treated my Mom well, and they loved each other, which was all that mattered. They had a bedroom in their house dedicated to him and (both of) their accolades. His albums and framed newspaper clippings hung on the walls.

One day, my cousin, who lived on the East Coast, called me and told me, "You need to go to Vegas and see what's going on with your mother!" Why? He said, "Things are disappearing off the walls." It sounded like he wasn't concerned about her but about "things" (dust). I called her and tried to speak with her on the phone, but she said, "Don't worry." I wrote her a letter and this time, unlike before, I sent it.

Dear Mama,

I am worried about you. Many people are worried about you, whether you want them to be or not. You don't get to choose who speaks about you because they love you.

As for myself, I am MORE worried about the fact that you refuse to be assessed or diagnosed and instead want to self-diagnose. In case you don't remember, you called me weeping at 8 a.m. one morning and begged me to come live with you. The next day, you had Don call me and tell me never to call your house again. I heard you in the background feeding him the words. I saved the message. And the next day, you called and said, "Hi baby, I haven't spoken to you in a while, so call me." Mom, I'm coming to visit!

So once again, I packed up Magic, his food and his litter box, and hit the road for Vegas. When I arrived, there were indeed gaping holes on the walls, where you could tell that items (Don's albums?) had been.

2017

March 25, 2017, Aunt Sheila passed away at 89

I knew I wouldn't return to New York for her funeral. I was extremely grateful that I had the presence of mind to visit her when she was alive and vital last year. After three strokes, her memory was gone, so I felt relief that she was finally at peace. I reached out to my cousins to share my grief. They understood why I couldn't make it back to sit shiva.

September 8

I wanted to be nearer to FDS and I really loved Fullerton. I was done with Long Beach. I needed out. I found a house in Fullerton, but with rent so high, I knew I needed a roommate. I found what looked like the perfect house, but little did I know that the roommate would turn out to be another bully in my life. Lucky me. She was a five-foot-nothing woman with a serious Napoleon complex. We didn't get off on the wrong foot initially, but over time, her personality became clear. She was a big rig truck driver and the daughter of the cantankerous man next door, who was the property's caretaker. To be fair, I later learned her father had dementia. That explained some of his erratic behavior. I thought the axiom "The apple doesn't fall far from the tree" had never been truer. I was validated, fortunately, when her lease ended. Our homeowner chose not to renew it. Instead, he offered me the chance to stay on my own—a blessing I gladly accepted. Knowing I could afford the place alone, I breathed a sigh of relief as she packed to leave. In response to one of her nasty notes about Magic, I wrote to her:

Napoleon complex: A short person who feels inferior because of their size. They tend to take it out on other people and thrive on power trips. Shouting at others, especially when they are in a position of power, was common. Side effects include short temper and anger issues. It is characterized by overly aggressive or domineering social behavior and implies that such behavior was compensatory for the subject's stature.

Take your pick of definitions. They all spell your name. The saddest part? You don't even see it. You said I should get help? Look in the mirror, lady. I have my family, friends, team, and church praying for you. I have all the support I need; you should get some. Again, focus on YOURself. My cat is none of YOUR business. Your reign of terror is over. Keep packing.

2018

Mom and I spoke regularly, which was nice—until things changed. She became belligerent, and I couldn't figure out why. She was 86, and her husband was 94. Some days, I would call her, and she was clear and coherent, and we had a lovely conversation. On other days, when I called, she was weeping or sobbing. For no apparent or obvious reason.

Sometimes, she would call and ask me for my phone number, leaving me confused and a bit unsettled. I wanted to say, "Mom, you just called me!" But I didn't. Other times, she would ask, "Who are you?" and when I replied, "It's Sheri," she would respond, "I have a daughter named Sheri." I had never dealt with dementia before, so I wasn't sure what to think. Once, she left me 30 to 40 voicemails in a single day. I took a screenshot, not for myself, but as proof that I needed to get a power of attorney in case anyone doubted the necessity. I said it before, hindsight is twenty-twenty. Looking back, I should have gotten conservatorship immediately.

I hated being so far away. I sent social workers to do a wellness check on her, and they came back with, "She's fine." Things had progressed from bad to worse, and she was anything but fine. When I hear the phrase "she's fine" or "you're fine," the bile rises in my throat. The kids say that a lot nowadays. I just look at them and think, "NOT fine!"

We spoke every couple of days or so. She mentioned she had a lady who worked at a nearby supermarket who was bringing them food and writing checks to pay their bills. I was horrified.

I had never been a parent. In my opinion, not having kiddos made me the perfect auntie! For anybody who had stayed awake nights trying to determine how to best care for their child, I was doing it now with my aging mama. Horrible to say, but my Mom was losing her marbles. To put it mildly, she was confused. The real indication that something was terribly wrong is that she stopped emailing and taking care of Don's website. She forgot how to use her laptop.

Things had gone from worse to even MORE worse. I'll be the first to admit we never had a perfect relationship, but at the end of the day, she's my Mom. I love her, I care about her, and I needed to take care of her. As her situation continued to worsen, I realized I had to act quickly. Getting a power of attorney (POA) became a priority, so I could make decisions in her best interests. I decided I would take care of her and her husband until the end of their lives. I did all my homework and found an attorney I wanted to use. I went to Vegas. I decided it was best to leave Magic home this trip. I left him a huge bowl of kibble and water. I told my neighbor what was going on, and asked her to please look in on him every couple of days. I packed some clothes and sped to Vegas. Luckily, I didn't get stopped or get a ticket. My heart was spinning, and my brain was filled with worry, not knowing what I would find.

When I arrived, everything seemed normal, whatever that meant. The only thing that disturbed me, the health nut, was that Mom and Don were eating ice cream sandwiches like they were going out of style. I had to beg them to stop eating the sugar.

They had four bags of asparagus in the fridge. Mom didn't cook, so I had no idea why that woman was bringing her things that needed cooking. I also discovered that she gave the key to her house to some dude, and I have no idea why. I didn't know if he was abusing her or stealing from her or what. Was that where the things off the wall went? There were so many ways Mom and Don could be taken advantage of; it wasn't even funny. I immediately made an appointment with their doctor to get an accurate assessment of them. When I asked her if she still exercised, she smiled and did a little dance—a plié followed by a pirouette. For a fleeting moment, her long-term memory surfaced, but it quickly slipped away, leaving a quiet sadness in the air which I inhaled with regret.

Since Don was in his nineties, I figured his memory was age-appropriate. He had heart issues, and I wasn't sure if Mom was giving him his meds appropriately. After their exams, due to privacy and HIPAA, the doctor was reluctant to share any results or diagnoses, even my Mom's. I told him I was her only child and beneficiary. It didn't matter to the doctor.

Next, it was time to assess their finances. We got out all her bills and bank and credit card statements. They were everywhere, in envelopes, paper bags and shoe boxes. I thought to myself - at least she had them! I wanted to get the bills online using autopay. More importantly, I needed to determine how much cash she had, where it was, and how long it would last to take care of her and Don. I prayed it would last until the end of their lives, whenever that would be. I did find a document from the doctor dated 2016 that said "possible dementia." I researched dementia on the internet. Then I thought, POSSIBLE?

I was texting with Don's daughter, who was willing to help. At one point we were trying to decide if we should have APS (Adult Protective Services) step in. She texted me:

"I made a lot of headway yesterday. When your mom left the room, my dad leaned over and said I was "the Francine whisperer". I wanted to die from laughter (every now and then my dad has these hilarious zingers) but I had to keep it in because I didn't want her to know what he said. I'm definitely more concerned about your mother than my dad. My only concern for my dad is her inability to remember even the simplest things. I went through the whole night time pill fiasco with her, and now that I've seen it, I get it. Her memory is so, so bad. All I could think about was "Finding Dory". Her memory works for minutes at a time now instead of the weeks and days as it used to be. Once I got firm, nice, but firm with her, she got scared. Not of me, but at the realization of what we already knew. My heart just broke for her. She remembers nothing of that conversation, I'm sure, but there was a definite moment of clarity there.

Here's where I want you to find comfort: I'm not just going to walk away and let someone else clean up the mess. Good or bad, they're our parents and the moral part of me is saying, "You can't just turn a blind eye to this even though they deserve none of my goodwill". Know that I'm going to treat your mom as if she were my own. Have they done a single thing to deserve any selflessness from us? Probably not. You and I follow the law of attraction, I also live under the law of karma. I'm no Mother Teresa, but I do what I feel is right. Am I making any sense?"

Yes she did make sense, but Don was declining quickly. He passed away shortly after I got there on April 4th. Every night after he passed, my Mom didn't sleep at all. She wandered around the house naked and would come into the room where I was (trying to) sleep and ask, "Where's Don?" I told her, "Mom, he passed away in your arms today."

The next night, the same thing happened, "Where's Don?" and I answered, "Mom, he passed away in your arms yesterday," then two days ago, then a week ago. This went on for weeks. I thought of the film *Groundhog Day*. I was living it. It was tragic. It was terrifying.

I planned to bring Mom to California to live with me, and I was sure I could get her better. I used to tell Ray, "Mama fix you," but now I needed to be her mama and say the same thing. I decided it was my turn to put my plans for my life aside and take care of her. She needed me. Living in her house without Don wasn't an option. I needed to sell her car and other things, pack her up, move her to California to live with me, and find us a house. So much to do.

I did a lot of research and discovered Dr. Bredesen, a doctor who was having great success halting and even reversing the symptoms of cognitive decline. I wanted to put her on Bredesen's protocol. I wanted to take her to my dentist. A lot of her caps were broken, and her beautiful mouth was in such disrepair that my heart broke seeing it. She said she was still driving her car, but I believe that was part of her confusion. I don't think she was driving, I had no idea. I just knew that she absolutely shouldn't be driving.

Things would change constantly as I tried to make plans for her and us—every minute, every hour, every day. She wanted to come to California with me, then she didn't. She wanted to be with her second cousins who also lived in Cali, then she didn't. Then, she was determined to go live with cousin in New York.

Meanwhile, cousin was p*ssing in her ear (excuse my bluntness, but there's no other way to put it), saying, "Well, you know how Sheri is." Maybe they knew how Sheri *was*, but Sheri wasn't a kid anymore. Mom had him on speaker, so I heard every word. When cousin and I spoke, he claimed he'd never take my Mom to New York.

After a month, I had to go home for my business, and make sure Magic was all right. I'd never been away from him before. I knew I couldn't leave Mom alone while I went back home, not even for a minute. One day, I caught her running around outside, half-dressed, lost, and confused. I called a friend who worked with me in my catering business. I knew she had caregiving experience. I bought her a plane ticket so she could fly to Vegas from Riverside, where she lived. After she arrived, I started my drive back home. Not even an hour later, Mom locked my friend and one of her friends out of the house. Really, Mom?

Thank God one of them had a phone on her and called me. I flipped a U-turn and sped back. I begged Mom to not do that again and to let these women be with her. She seemed to be accepting, so once again, I got in my car and got on the road.

After two weeks, I returned to Vegas. Cousin was calling every day. I begged him to come and help me, but he said he was unable. He finally told me and admitted he lost his driver's license, so he couldn't get on a plane. I started making plans to sell her car and all her possessions. Then, at cousin's urging, Mom's second cousins came from Cali and started doing the very things I had been trying to do for her—cataloging her stuff and planning next steps. I was stunned. Wow. I guess I was no longer needed. Cousin was calling constantly, directing them on what to do and how to do it, while I watched from the sidelines. I thought: time to go.

When you fly on an airplane, the flight attendant instructs you to "put your oxygen mask on first" before helping others with theirs. Why is this an important rule for ensuring survival? If you run out of oxygen yourself, you can't help anyone else. I had to survive. I had to walk away. I hated having to do so. I knew, in my heart, I was not going to give up.

We continued speaking on the phone. One day, she wanted to live with me, and the next day she wanted to go to New York and live with cousin. I was torn, but always hopeful. I knew I could fix her. She took care of me for the first 15 years of my life, and I wanted to care for her during her last 15 years or however much time she would live.

I found out her cousins were able to get conservatorship, but then cousin in NY harassed them so horribly that they had to leave as well. I don't know what happened after that. I called her HOA to get info on what was going on. The lady said cousin and his wife were living in Mom's house and refurbishing it. I figured if he was caring for her and keeping her safe, so be it. I just wanted to hear her voice so badly it hurt.

Once again, I asked my doctor for something to help with my anxiety and sleepless nights.

When I got back to California, I took an APOE gene test and a MOCA test (the Montreal Cognitive Assessment), a tool for early detection of mild cognitive impairment (MCI). So many people have told me they wouldn't want to know. Can you spell ostrich? My APOE results came back as e3/e3, meaning an estimated 10-15% risk of developing MCI by age 85, and an 85-90% chance of not developing it. My MOCA score was 26 out of 30, though I suspect my nerves caused me to score so low!

Not a day went by that I didn't think about Ray, dwell on his memory, or shed tears over losing him. His ashes were always with me— around my neck, beside my bed, and in my car. His image surrounded me too, with screensavers and photos of him in every room. I even bought a stainless steel chain to wear his ashes, along with my Navy dog tag and my dad's Army dog tag. His ashes are in a beautiful stainless tube gifted to me by Dr. J when he ran his Ashes to

Ashes business. The biggest lesson I've learned from animals tearing off my necklace in the past was that since dog tags are irreplaceable I wasn't going to risk losing them by having a traditional chain.

2019

January 21

I had booked a few events that wanted a chocolate fountain, so I subcontracted with a company that specialized in them. Then I thought - why keep subcontracting when I could do this just as well, if not better? It turned out the owner was looking to sell her business so she could spend more time with her children. It felt like the perfect opportunity. I thought this would be the year I'd finally get ahead.

Meditation was helping me become more mindful. As I looked around, I realized everything God had placed in my life was a blessing. I made sure to give thanks. I tried to focus on letting go of the guilt. Guilt about my success and about walking away from my Mom. But the truth was, I missed her like crazy. I thought about her every single day. My heart ached for her, and soon, that worry turned inward. I didn't want fear to consume me, but I didn't know how to stop it. I even considered asking Dr. Bredesen if "hysterical empathy" existed.

March

Dr. Bredesen was attending NPE, and somehow, I always knew I'd meet him. Intuition? Wishful thinking? I reached out to him on LinkedIn, and to my shock, he accepted my request to connect. I'd long admired his groundbreaking work in cognitive decline—he'd had remarkable success stopping and even reversing it. I desperately wanted to put Mom on his protocol; I had always held onto hope that I could "fix" her. But how could I do that when I didn't even know where she was?

Despite cousin swearing he'd never take Mom in, I later heard she was with him. The moment I found out, I pictured her with him, despite his firm declaration: "I will NEVER have your mom with me in New York." I wasn't sure what changed, but I couldn't bring myself to ask him. Why bother? He lied.

I got a letter from the Hawaii Supreme Court's Disciplinary Board about the attorney whose incompetence cost me my house. Five years later, they finally sent a letter telling me they'd given him a disciplinary warning. Big woo. Too little, too late.

The 2020s

January

It was the start of a new decade, and I stayed optimistic that someday I'd be with my Mom. How? I hadn't a clue. I just held onto that optimism. I had to. When people asked how she was, I couldn't answer, and I couldn't say why I couldn't answer.

I called both of cousin's sons, trying to track her down. Both said they hadn't spoken to their dad in over five years. They said that he was a horrible human and couldn't help me. One said that he heard through the grapevine that my Mom was in a nursing home in the Bronx. The grapevine? Really? Nevertheless, I was determined to call every single one to find her. I started compiling a list of all the nursing homes in the Bronx, but the task was daunting. There were a ton, and that is an understatement. Plus, no one bothered to answer the phone or return calls or messages. Thank you, pandemic.

The bottom line was that I could not speak with her for years. My poor Mommy, I thought of her constantly. Trying to imagine what it was like to be without memory. I put a picture of her up on the wall in my garage, so I'd see it every day when I pulled in. Each time I pulled in, I whispered a prayer for her. Louise Hay, in *101 Power Thoughts for Life*, wrote, "Put something beautiful up so when you come home …"

I finally got the digital copy of my M&M commercial! It was proof that persistence pays off. That, and a refusal to take no for an answer. I had to fight with the Mars Company for years.

They tried to say they couldn't let me see it or have a copy as it was a legal issue. I countered with, "It's MY likeness." I hounded them to let me have a digital copy. My doggedness paid off. I won! They sent it to me, and I put it on my YouTube channel. It was too late for Aunt Sheila to see it, but I hoped one day I could show it to my Mom. I knew she would get a kick out of seeing it again after so many years.

J was still in jail, probably preaching to inmates just like he had at the flophouse. Was he taking his meds? I'd never know. And that was just fine. I forgave him because he is sick. How could one not forgive someone's behavior if it is due to mental illness? The pity was that he was sentenced to ten years, and they released him after just three. Then, they put him back in jail. VINE notified me every time something happened due to the restraining order. If I had to guess, probably because he stopped using the meds that helped him and returned to his bad behavior. People with bipolar disorder often think, "I feel fine; I don't need meds anymore." WRONG!

March

Henry's mother was dealing with some medical drama, so he took on the responsibility of caring for her. He told me he'd had enough of catering and was ready to retire. He was my age, how could I blame him? At least he owned his kitchen and would be able to. I was freaking out just a little.

PP said she would execute my events. She *knew* I was freaking out. She had no desire to do this, but again, it's just the type of person and friend she is. She is also a writer. She wrote a book, *Food Fun Love Party Styles*, and gave me a copy when it was released. Loved it! Then she wrote another book, a memoir entitled *My Culinary Love Story*, and gave me a copy of that as well. Loved it!! I let her read my screenplay. I guess she thought it was decently written, that perhaps I had talent. She asked me to adapt the second book into a screenplay (gulp).

Then, the pandemic hit. Panic spread faster than the virus. A sign on the bank door read: "No hats. No sunglasses. No hoodies." No mention of masks. A great time to be a bank robber.

When everyone was freaking out about not having toilet paper, there was a full case on my shelf. Let's just say no one could ever accuse me of being a procrastinator.

With the world on pause, I threw myself into my passions—cooking, writing, creating. Anything to distract my mind. Since moving into this house in 2017, I'd had a garage full of boxes and decided it was finally time to unpack them. What does a caterer do during a pandemic when there are no events? Feed the homeless. Maybe I couldn't help Mom, but I could help someone. That had to count for something.

God directed me to the Rock Church. The Food Bank was delivering a ton of food in bulk, so they needed volunteers to separate and bag it for individual households. We did that all week, and then on Saturday, we gave them out.

No matter what I did, no matter how busy I kept myself, my thoughts always drifted back to Mom. Was she safe? Was she scared? I constantly wondered how she was doing.

June 22

I found this post on FB: #CondemnTheCastle.

Dear Lower Puna,

We have a VERY serious issue in our community that has a very easy solution if we all take five minutes. The infamous "Castle" in Seaview has become a total drug den of meth and heroin users. Ten to twenty meth and heroin abusers live there at a time. More are coming because the word on the street is the Castle is the spot to live free and stay on drugs! There are known rapists, pedophiles, and murderers that pass through this place.

This Castle is a total hotbed for EVERY kind of infectious disease, including COVID-19. There are rumors that peeps living there have severe respiratory illnesses but won't go to hospital due to drug addiction. However, they will hang out at Kehena all day, making a scene. These drugged-out zombies have now started wandering Seaview and Red Road to steal for their next hit. Residents have had a noticeable increase in meth heads roaming around carports and houses. They are routinely seen on the lawn and beach having whacked-out conversations with themselves in their drug-induced minds.

Numerous women have had super scary encounters. Two near rapes happened right at the tsunami/wedding point location across from Kalani. I will spare the real horror stories of the underage trafficking I heard has happened there. Some local Hawaiians have warned them, and police have visited, but it hasn't made the issue go away at all.

So, finally, a group of locals have come up with a simple, peaceful, legal, legit solution. If the city legally condemns the Castle, then the police can legally vacate the house, and we can board it up so this plague doesn't come back.

The owner, Castle J, is in jail, and the wife is gone, so it's basically a squatted structure. There is NO ELECTRICITY OR RUNNING WATER, and yet 10-20 drug addicts live there? This is a legit building to condemn legally. Right now, police can't do much since everyone can just leave and then return and claim they don't live there.

However, if the County condemns the building, they must leave! I have already contacted the City and filed a report of the building code violations a week ago, but I haven't heard back. If anyone would like to join and help us, PM letting us know what you can offer. All help is appreciated. I will be posting our next meeting so anyone can attend, and we are going to take action if the county doesn't.

Needless to say, nothing was done. Why am I not surprised? Still, "Welcome to Hawaii" after all these years. The place was covered in mold when I left. Let the squatters figure out what that does to a body. Karma's got it handled.

End of 2020

I missed my Mom terribly. I had a brainstorm. J would have said, "Treat it kindly, it's in a strange place." I called Mom's dear friend of 60 years in NY. Her daughter and I had been best friends back in the sixties, and to my surprise, her number was still the same. Even more amazing, she picked up the phone when I called! She was 88, and still sharp. I told her what was going on, that I'd been trying to find Mom for years since Don died, and that Mom lost her marbles.

I asked her to call cousin and see if he would give her Mom's location or number to call her. She called him. Thank goodness, he couldn't say no to her. He told her that Mom was living with a caregiver named Julie on Long Island. Then he added, "Don't give the info to Sheri." Seriously? What I heard in my head was "Don't tell Sheri." She called the number cousin gave her, and spoke to Mom. She immediately called me afterwards and gave me the number. She said Mom had remembered her. That was good to hear and surprising, but it made me happy.

I called immediately and had a long conversation with Julie. Her first question caught me off guard: "You're not going to take your mom from me, are you?" I was incredulous. Why would I do that? It made me wonder if cousin had threatened her. Later, I learned that he was paying her $6,000 a month for Mom to live with her. Then, when #CovidCrap happened, he decided to reduce the payment to $4,000. That didn't make any sense. What did COVID have to do with caregiving?

No matter, I was FINALLY able to speak with her. I was ecstatic! I called her every day. I mailed her cards and pictures. Julie emailed me a picture of her. She got Mom's hair done. Although Mom seemed a bit dazed (zombie-like) in the picture, on the whole, she was alive. I was grateful for the picture, and for the ability to speak to her. Julie seemed to care about her and take good care of her, which brought me some comfort, but what would happen if or after Mom passed? Especially if she were in New York. She wanted to be buried next to her husband in Vegas; they had plots next to each other.

October 23 is Mom's birthday. I called to wish her a happy one! This day, when I called, Julie said, "Your mom's not here." What do you mean she's not there? My heart dropped, thinking the worst.

"Your cousin came and took her," she said. She didn't know where he took her. What could I say? The joy of finally speaking with her had been fleeting. Once again, he ripped it away.

Every time the news mentioned "prophylactics" for Covid, my mind went somewhere else entirely. Haven't thought about it in a while. Haven't had any in a while. Ten years? Fifteen years? Get over it. I think to myself: you had enough when you were young. Payback's a bitch. I must say I miss cuddling and having my back scratched. Can a person suddenly become asexual? I looked it up since I looked up everything. Wiki says: Asexuality is the lack of sexual attraction to others or low or absent interest in, or desire for, sexual activity. Question answered.

For years, I hauled a trunk from coast to coast, stuffed with every letter ever written to me—a treasure trove of memories dating back to the '60s. These letters capture moments in time, serving as a window into my life and the relationships that have shaped it, preserving both personal history and cultural shifts across decades. There were a ton from Mom, Nat and George. It was very cool and thought-provoking to revisit them.

I decided to scan everything, and as I worked through the collection, I found myself laughing and reminiscing over each one. Many of the people who wrote these letters are still in my life today. I published them and called the series *When We Wrote Letters*. A **biography** is a detailed account of a person's life written by someone else. It typically includes significant events, achievements, experiences, and personal details, often providing insights into the person's character, relationships, and impact on the world. So it's a biography. Given the extensive collection, I chose to organize it into books by decade. The letters from the '60s and '70s were so abundant I had to split them into two volumes. I felt there were simply too many pages to fit into a single book.

As I sifted through the letters, I was struck by how many names I didn't recognize. Why didn't people include last names? Dates? Something! Whether anyone will care to read them is yet to be seen, but I'll self-publish these books nonetheless. This project is more than a biography—it's a time capsule of voices from the past, capturing moments that feel both personal and universal. It's a love letter to the people and places that shaped me, to a time that feels both distant and just yesterday.

I bought a lottery ticket, not for myself, but for the joy of sharing—just as Kabbalah teaches. I created a list of everyone in my life to whom I wanted to give a cash gift. I wanted to make foundations for ALZ, ALS, cancer, autism, animal rescue, and more causes. I felt a compelling desire to do good in the world. I often wondered what the lottery winners did with the money they won. I heard horror stories that some lost everything and were worse off than when they started a few years later.

When I pass a homeless encampment, in the back of my mind, I know God is trying to remind me to do what is tugging at my heart and be involved in trying to make housing for un-housed people. I discovered Mobile Loaves and Fishes (mlf.org) in Austin, and I am obsessed with wanting something similar here in all the

SoCal counties: OC (Orange County), then in LA County, Riverside, San Diego County, and San Gabriel. I am determined to try to do something about the homeless situation. I know God will give me directions and strength. Living without a roof over your head must be the most horrible thing imaginable. There but for the grace of God. That is one of the first things I will set aside money for out of lottery winnings. Especially for the veterans.

I want to do the same thing with Marama. Marama is a dementia care community founded by Dr. Heather Sandison in San Diego, California. It was designed as a fully immersive residential care facility that integrates the Bredesen Protocol—a multi-modal approach aimed at reversing cognitive decline. The facility is focused on holistic care, providing organic, keto-flex meals, non-toxic living environments, and brain-healing activities to support residents in their journey to better cognitive health. Marama's mission is to not only improve but potentially reverse the effects of Alzheimer's and dementia through comprehensive lifestyle changes and cutting-edge interventions. There needs to be one in every county! And I want to buy all my friends a Toyota Mirai—no emissions! It uses hydrogen fuel.

After six years back in SoCal, I was finally thinking about adopting a dog—maybe a tiny one, a pocket pup. I was lonely and missing my Mom, and I thought getting a dog would help.

My thoughts turned to Bruiser, our sausage. We'd gotten him when he was just six weeks old. When J went to prison, he left poor Bruiser, already eight or nine years old by then, with strangers. How traumatic that must have been for Bruiser, being abandoned by his daddy. Even though I forgave J for everything he perpetrated against me, I think the only thing I would never forgive him for is not letting me have Bruiser when he went to jail. One day, Daniel messaged me on Facebook: Bruiser had a seizure and died. Huh? He was only 12. He'd never been sick a day in his life. He should have had at least three or four more years.

I searched the internet rescue sites for "Dachshund" and all I came up with were dogs that were mixed. Not one looked like a real Doxie. The day after thinking about this, I ran into a woman holding a Chihuahua at Petco. I asked her if I could meet her little guy. She said he wasn't hers. A homeless man walked away from him, so she just grabbed him. He was very grabbable, I must say. She started whining about how she couldn't keep him, as dogs weren't allowed where she lived.

I looked at this dog, he looked at me, and suddenly, I felt Ray. I imagined Ray was reincarnated in this animal. Intuition or just wishful thinking? I told her I would take him, and she happily handed him over with relief. He was itchy and scratchy. I figured he was infested with fleas since he was a homeless dog, and I was correct.

The minute we got home, I put him in the kitchen sink and bathed him. He wasn't a fan. Then we raced to the vet to get him checked out. The vet asked what his name was, and since

I couldn't think of anything original, I blurted out, "Bruiser." The vet put flea medication on him, and then Bruiser II and I went back home to get acquainted. I posted on FB: "In a perfect world, every dog would have a home, and every home would have a dog."

Bruiser (II) is the closest thing I've had to a real baby. This tiny Chihuahua is every bit the two-year-old toddler. If you ask him if he wants food or water, even if he is starving or thirsty, he puts his nose in the air and turns his head away. He could be famished, but he will sniff the food and walk away. Then he returned a few minutes later and ate. I cracked up about that. Magic did the same thing.

I reconnected with my friend Lydia. She used to come to the castle and bring amazing, outrageous, wonderful, delightful, delicious cookie dough, and we would bake cookies with her dough and watch movies. We called each other "cookie face." She had returned to California a little while before I did. It turned out she had ovarian cancer, and her outlook on health was much like mine. She told me she'd had surgery to remove it but refused chemo or radiation, unwilling to put poison in her body. I would feel the same—prioritizing quality of life above all else.

She's a little younger than me, and she is experiencing the same effects of aging: dry eye, lack of sleep or being able to sleep, and peeing constantly. She came and I made her dinner. We commiserated. We shared our latest health discoveries. She brought Sandy, her senior Golden Retriever. Sandy and Bruiser (II) became instant buddies. Both were terrified of fireworks, so we made it a tradition to spend the Fourth of July together.

We stayed in my bedroom, closed the window, cranked up the air conditioner and blasted the TV.

In my mind? Once you reach 60 years of age, it's all downhill. Suddenly, seemingly, one day, everything changes. Everything becomes more difficult. Clothes are more difficult to put on and take off; jars are more difficult to open.

When I was flying back and forth from Hawaii to the mainland, tossing a fifty-pound suitcase around was no big deal—it was just part of the routine. Now? A thirty-pound package feels like I'm trying to lift the weight of the world. Funny how things change and how gravity seems to get stronger as the years go by! After talking to friends, I realized I wasn't alone in this.

My eyes changed. It's more difficult to see. Plus, my eyes are sandy and gritty. I went to the eye doctor, who diagnosed dry eye. I'd never heard of it. When he recommended that I put a hot compress on my eyes every morning, my first reaction was, "Yeah, that'll never happen." Trust me, it happens if you don't want to be miserable all day. And even then, sometimes I do it multiple times a day. And put in artificial tears multiple times a day. I researched prescription medication, but the price was prohibitive. One of them costs $600 a month. It started in March 2020 when #CovidCrap first started. "They" said, "Don't put your hands near your eyes." Ha ha. "They" never had dry eye. Someone told me to use a humidifier. I got two. That's just the kind of gal I am.

I noticed my hairline was receding, and much of my hair was falling out. I referred to it as shedding, like a cat or dog. I started buying everything I could find to try to stave it off. I think swimming aggravated it with all the chlorine in the water.

Another fabulous condition I noticed is that my skin had gotten paper-thin. If I bump into something, I get a huge red blotch. Not a black-and-blue mark, but a horrible, ugly blotch.

The top of my feet started to hurt. I tried to ignore it, but the pain grew worse and worse. I noticed a lump or cyst or something growing on the top of the left one. I decided to go to a podiatrist and have it checked out since I have Medicare and don't have to pay for doctor visits now. (That might be the *only* good thing about growing old.) The podiatrist took an x-ray and found out it was arthritis. Bone on bone. My right knee had surgery 20 or so years ago. Now, it needs to be replaced. Bone on bone. My left knee isn't happy, but not as bad … yet. My left shoulder started popping, then hurting. Back to ortho. Bone on bone. My right shoulder isn't happy, but not as bad … yet.

I don't eat for flavor; I focus on healthy ingredients. Sometimes, the taste might not be great, but that's not what matters to me. I still finish every bite. I've had this mindset since I was 16, when I first became a "health nut." I don't eat traditional breakfast foods either. I prefer protein to fuel my morning, rather than starting my day (like a lot of people) with donuts or toast and jams, and orange juice - too much sugar!

I've never been able to eat before noon or 1 p.m. Apparently, this is now a "thing," called intermittent fasting, which is extremely good for brain health. You aren't supposed to eat until 12 hours or more after your last meal the previous night. Everything changes, doesn't it? Make coffee with cold water; no need. Freeze coffee, don't freeze. Eggs are bad for you; eggs are good for you. Make hard-boiled eggs in cold water to start. No, boil water and then put the eggs in. Make up my mind.

Sometimes, the world is too much to bear. I imagine trying to get it over with, if you will, but I think I'm too big of a chicken. Tomorrow is not promised; we all die. We all suffer. I miss Ray so much. I miss my mama. Suck up. I tell myself: "Put on your big girl panties."

What do you want on your tombstone? *If* I wanted a tombstone, which I do not, I would like it to read: "Susie Sunshine Sleeps Here." I don't want to be buried; I don't want to be burned. I donated my body to science. I want some young doctor to use it to learn and make the world better. I found out you can't just say you want to donate your body; you must execute paperwork to do so. After doing some online research, I realized UCLA fit the bill perfectly.

I want to be a ray of positivity and light when I call or connect! RAY of positivity, see what I did there? The sea of awareness. I jumped in! What a tremendous concept. It's one of those ideas that, once you see it, you can't unsee it. It changes everything. I don't understand why people call each other names; it's such a waste when we could be swimming in the sea of awareness instead.

Grief is a horrible word. How does one deal with it? In my opinion, we don't "move on" from grief; we move forward with it. When you lose a beloved, you gain an organ that secretes sadness for the rest of your life. Even though my mama is not dead, I'm secreting this sadness for her now also, as well as my boy.

I don't want a celebration of life, but if I did, I'd want my favorite songs played. Especially those I played for Ray. Especially when I need a good cry:

1. Good Things Fall Apart by Jon Bellion ("I guess that sometimes good things fall apart.")

2. See You Again by Charlie Puth ("It's been a long day without you, my friend And I'll tell you all about it when I see you again. Why'd you have to leave me when I needed you the most?")

3. Say Something by A Great Big World ("Anywhere, I would've followed you.") and

4. Ho Hey by - the Lumineers ("I belong with you, you belong with me you're my sweet…")

I am grateful for everything and am mindful to be so. The one thing I am the most grateful for? Discovering meditation. I try to meditate and swim every single day. If I do not meditate or swim every day, I know it. I feel anxious and uncomfortable.

Thank you @DanBHarris, for Ten Percent Happier, which has made a profound difference in my life, and I am glad to proclaim it and give credit where credit is due. I found it curious how many meditation teachers, particularly those with Jewish backgrounds, have embraced Buddhism and wonder what drew them to this path. I want to be a teacher; this may be my life's purpose. I feel that teaching isn't just about sharing knowledge; it's about inspiring growth, fostering curiosity, and helping people realize their potential. The chance to guide and support others deeply aligns with my life's purpose.

I'm also grateful for the Calm app. I get up two to four times a night to pee, after which I listen to a sleep story. If I do not, I spin for the rest of the night. The first time I tried it, I thought: "Listen to a bedtime story? What am I, three years old?" So many things I never thought I could do, but I now do.

I am also grateful for three podcasts. There are so many of them that when I find one worth listening to, I start at the beginning and listen to every single episode. The first one was *Ten Percent Happier.* The second was *The Empowering Neurologist.* Dr. Perlmutter has educated me extensively, especially about dementia and Alzheimer's. The third one was *Love Conquers Alz*, produced by Susie Singer Carter. Fun fact: I connected with her in 2018 when I was first marketing PeopleMakePlans.com. I pitched to her. She passed. Oh well, so did a bunch of others. But then I got wind of a short film she made called *My Mom and the Girl,* starring Valerie

Harper, and it was phenomenal. I became a rabid fan. When I discovered her podcast, I listened to every episode.

I do not believe that when you stand before your maker, you will be asked, "How much money did you make down there?" Rather, "What good did you do?" If I hear "You're too nice" one more time, I swear I'll lose it. I tell them I live Aloha, and it's not just a word; it's a way of life. When you are mindful and treat others as you wish to be treated, you find the law of attraction working, and you will connect with other like-minded individuals. For a long while, I was attracting abuse, and when I became mindful about it, it stopped. Or I stopped it. When I think of something, and it suddenly appears, I am mindful to give thanks.

When someone says, "You made me …" I say, "I don't *make* you *anything*." I learned this important fact when I studied NVC (nonviolent communication), which was one of the few things J introduced me to that was positive. We studied NVC and Kabbalah, as we tried to get along and learn how to live with each other.

I drink too much. Maybe not by some standards, but for me? One glass feels like one too many. Not because I'm hungover. I *am* dehydrated, but that's a quick fix. Yet I keep doing it and hate myself the next day. And still, I don't stop. I am now aware it's bad for the brain. I learned that after all my research on dementia following time with Mom. I discovered on Dr. Perlmutter's podcast just how bad drinking is for the brain. But when it's five o'clock, I crave just 6-8 ounces of red wine. My reward for surviving another day on this rock.

I always knew that "white" foods—sugar, rice, and the like—weren't great for you. But Dr. Perlmutter introduced me to a healthier alternative for sweetening (especially my coffee!) that might even have benefits: allulose. Recent studies provided insights into the potential health benefits of allulose, a rare sugar that is lower in calories and has a minimal effect on blood glucose levels.

When a family member is diagnosed with dementia, the fear of facing it yourself becomes hard to ignore. You start questioning every moment of forgetfulness, like walking into a room and forgetting why you're there. Robin Williams' tragic suicide after his diagnosis of Lewy Body Dementia brought this frightening disease into the public eye. Bruce Willis' diagnosis with Frontotemporal Dementia (FTD) has given another face to these debilitating conditions. Seeing someone so larger-than-life reduced by this disease is heartbreaking. It forces us all to confront our own fragility.

Thankfully, his family has been open about his journey, sharing real, firsthand experiences that help educate others about what living with dementia truly means. That transparency is invaluable, offering hope and understanding, but it doesn't erase the anxiety of knowing how devastating these illnesses can be.

2021

In my ideal world, the moment I get up after having a wonderful night's sleep of seven to eight hours without having to pee two to three times (ha-ha). The "youngins" nowadays call this is a workflow. My schedule/flow would be:

1. Drink two tablespoons of apple cider vinegar or take a shot of extra virgin olive oil (EVOO). It is VERY challenging—neither is known for

its yummy taste! Both are known for health benefits, especially for the brain.

2. Put a hot compress on my eyes, put eye drops in my eyes.

3. Watch the news because one must have a daily dose of fear, doesn't one? (Tongue in cheek.)

4. Use the low-light laser I used on Ray's spine for his lumbar stenosis on my receding hairline and my wrinkles. Voodoo? AND do this at night while watching my comedies.

5. Use Minoxidil or something similar on my receding hairline. Or do this at night while watching my comedies.

6. Use a ton of moisturizer on the wrinkles on my face. Or use the newest miracle cream that promises to get rid of wrinkles. That's a joke. None of them do. AND do this at night before watching my comedies. Lately, I've

been using a micro-needler to see if that would help.

7. Eat a little something while being mindful of intermittent fasting so I could take my handful of vitamins and supplements. Then take a memory supplement. It *was* Prevagen or Neuriva, which were way too expensive. Plus, I found out they didn't work despite the testimonials promising they did. Now, I'm trying another supplement with a 365-day return policy. We'll see. I also take these supplements (for brain and on an empty stomach): phosphatidylserine, and acetyl-L-carnitine. Turmeric, ginkgo biloba, cinnamon and red yeast rice for brain and high cholesterol.

8. Meditate and do Paraliminals.

9. Clean cat litter boxes.

10. Go to the gym to swim, workout with weights, or take a class. I don't have to

pay for my gym anymore. Medicare pays for silver sneakers. That's the ONLY other good thing about getting old.

I made lists of what I wanted to do but trying to do everything I wanted to do was extremely time-consuming. At some point, it just seemed like too much trouble, took too long, or other things came up diverting my attention. Some days, I tackled it all like a warrior. Other days? The best I could do was brush my teeth and call it a win.

It's interesting to reflect on how little was known about bipolar disorder back in the '90s. J and I kept a diary, and reading it now, it's painfully obvious that I had no clue what was happening. I just thought he was "insane." Scanning and publishing that diary felt like a way to help others deal with the disorder, but it also served as a window into our past struggles. Reading it years later, it's obvious to me that what I once labeled as madness was really the result of an untreated illness. That understanding was why I was able to forgive him.

After the January 6th Capitol riots, I visited a gun store to explore purchasing a lady gun, inquire about prices, and sign up for shooting lessons. I wanted to find out how much it would cost. In the back of my mind, I worried about shooting myself in the foot. A man standing behind me in line suggested wasp spray. The salesperson behind the counter gave him stink eye. I decided that was a much better option for me. I bought three cans and keep one by my bedroom door, the front door, and the back door—just in case someone decided to invade my home. That is what I wanted a gun for, not to carry around with me. Problem solved in a much better way!

I watch too much news. Living alone in a vacuum, I try to get different perspectives on what's happening in the world. One thing I know for sure is that I keep my opinions to myself. I don't post publicly on Facebook, Instagram, or elsewhere. These days, it's too easy for people to snipe at one another and offer opinions that nobody asked for.

I should clarify—I *do* post to promote the chocolate fountain business, but nothing personal. The only drama I want online is melted chocolate cascading down a fountain.

Meanwhile, I see people sharing their shiny lives, sending happy birthday or anniversary wishes through social media. Pick up the phone! I'm sure they'd much rather hear your voice than read a post, don't you think?

It drives me crazy when people post and disclose their medical information online! A friend once asked me why I feel that way. I think sharing that kind of personal detail is like handing criminals—especially hackers and scammers—ammunition to exploit you.

For the first time in my life, I don't have my earnings/money snatched out of my hand by a bully. Granted, we were moving toward a goal and trying to finish our castle. However, it was disconcerting when I wasn't asked how I would like to spend the money I earned. I think the only question I was asked was what color I wanted the walls in the bedroom to be.

Confusion is a horrible thing. Cognitive decline is awful. Everybody says f*ck cancer. I say f*ck bipolar, f*ck Alzheimer's, f*ck dementia, f*ck ALS (Lou Gehrig's disease), AND f*ck cancer double. When I got skin cancer, how could I be surprised since I went on the roof of the buildings in Manhattan in the 8th, 9th, and 10th grades to get a suntan with a sun reflector and baby oil? All the girls in my school did.

Living in Hawaii for 15 years was my dress rehearsal for understanding the importance of community. On the Big Island, failing to foster strong relationships with neighbors could have life-or-death consequences, especially with tsunamis, hurricanes, and lava flows potentially cutting off essential resources like water and food. Similarly, with the chaos of the #CovidCrap back on the mainland, building a sense of community has become vital for survival, whether with hundreds of people or simply your immediate neighbors. I feel blessed to live in a safe cul-de-sac surrounded by wonderful, kind neighbors.

We have each other's phone numbers and look out for one another.

I haven't been sick in ten years. As soon as I even "think" I have a bug, I run for the kombucha. I get three vitamin Cs and take one (1000 mg.) every six hours. Out comes the arsenal of homeopathic drops in the fridge: oregano, rosemary, olive leaf, echinacea and goldenseal, and maitake mushroom. Elderberry extract is next. Then garlic, garlic, garlic. Did I mention garlic? I roast a whole head. Low and slow in a pocket of tin foil, smothered in olive oil. Then use the olive oil for cooking or salad dressing.

I don't normally eat bread, but I go for sourdough, pumpernickel, or rye if I do. Then the bread goes into the toaster with a big clove of soft, roasted garlic smeared on it. Then I run to a place that squeezes wheatgrass juice and buy two ounces. I have a juicer, but it's easier to buy. The average person should start with one ounce or be close to the restroom.

I spoke to a lady who assists people with Medicare to ensure they have the correct coverage. I mentioned in passing that I suffered from dry eye. She suggested I visit a nearby doctor who makes eye drops from your blood serum. I did, and nine months later, my eyes were so incredibly improved I could barely believe it. Thanks, Deb!

April 4

I fostered two German shepherds, which was ironic since I swore I would never own another GSD. The universe has a twisted sense of humor. But really, I meant one of my own. We connected on dogsondeployment.org. Their dad had to deploy on a submarine, and he had nowhere to leave them. He thought he would have to give them up. How could I say no?

Unfortunately for the dogs, military service comes before training dogs. Jasmine was three, and Max was four. These two had no training to speak of. They barked and barked and barked. They were like an old married couple! The one thing I know for sure is you must wear your dog out, so I bought a heavy-duty mobility scooter.

I figured I could sell it when they left. I cannot run or even walk for long due to my wobbly knee that needs replacement. They were crated at night, and I'd never been a fan of this practice, but these guys needed it. They barked crazy loud for the first 20 minutes when I went out and said hello in the morning, then I took them out for a jog. My neighbor in the house next to the kennels hated me.

August 8

How can it be that the minute the pandemic kinda sorta ended, my pre-pandemic life returned as well? God is great and knows what we need better than we do, from having an abundance overload and being able to feed homeless people and help friends. Back to trying to manifest catering jobs, making connections on LinkedIn, trying to get a development deal for People Make Plans, sending out emails for catering, waking at 4, 5, or 6 a.m., and never having enough time to do everything each day.

I got the flu shot every year, and after Whoopi and Oprah got pneumonia and almost died, I started getting the pneumonia vaccine, even though I haven't been sick in forever. I have never gotten measles, mumps, or chickenpox (which I always called chicken pops when I was a child) or any of the usual childhood diseases.

Nowadays, every time you turn around, somebody's trying to shove a needle in your arm for shingles or whatever else they are selling. Since I haven't had chickenpox, I will probably never get shingles, thank God. How many vaccines can a person put in their body? The only needle I put in my body is a vitamin B12 shot. And I do that myself once a month. Glad I learned the proper way when I was in the Navy.

I asked Producer Jeff, my hānai son, to revise and improve People Make Plans. Being too close to the story was hindering me. Plus, my knowledge about structure can fit on the head of a thimble. WHEN it sells, I will give him "written with" credit.

JoJo's favorite pastime is playing cards, and she's taught me a bunch of games. No one writes letters or plays cards anymore except perhaps me and JoJo.

After Gummy died, he told me to "watch out for her." Yes, *after* he died. I knew he was still with me! Another example of my uniqueness? I think that is why the law of attraction introduced me to Char.

WHAT DO I WANT MY LEGACY TO BE?

How do I want to be remembered? In interviews on TV, the reporter always seems to ask people that question. This is what I want mine to be:

She had a sharp wit and self-deprecating humor, much like Dan Harris, founder of *Ten Percent Happier*. She had a big heart but no patience for stupidity. She always wanted to help people and share her knowledge, especially regarding health and supplements. She was funny and could make people laugh. She was kind and had integrity. She was generous with her time and resources. She was truly magnanimous.

Kabbalah teaches money is energy. What can you hope to accomplish or acquire if you are a schnorrer (Jewish term for cheapskate)? Not much, in my experience. According to Kabbalah, there is no difference between a penny on the ground or a billion dollars in the bank or a hundred-dollar bill in your hand, for that matter. If you believe what Kabbalah teaches, you know that it's all dust, and the only thing we have is love and our relationships. I am acutely aware of receiving for the self alone, trying to live the principles of Kabbalah. If I want blessings, I know I must give selflessly, even when it hurts, especially when it hurts. J once said: "Once you are made aware of precepts," he was speaking of Mormonism, "You have no choice but to live by them."

Being on an island in Hawaii, it was important to keep things local. I believed in keeping it local even before I went to Hawaii. Translated in my world: I believe in being loyal. If somebody is doing a good job for you, keep using them.

I have always been #GirlBoss. However, now I know how to do it with integrity without pissing off everyone I come into contact with, like I used to. Hopefully, I'm doing it successfully. I immediately noticed how people react when I walk around with a smile on my face. Even when I don't feel like smiling, I do it anyway—it starts to feel less forced over time, and the positive reactions make it worth it.

September 28

Every time I plan out a day, I mindfully consider the best use of my time. Tuesday is Panera bread donation day. I head to the parks to distribute food and other stuff (blankets, clothes, etc.) I collect. But now that the pandemic has pretty much ended, I don't have time or resources to keep driving around in my big, beautiful, gas-guzzling van searching for homeless people.

People throw around words so carelessly—empty promises, vague commitments, plans that never materialize. "Say what you mean, mean what you say" isn't just a cliché; it's a basic principle of respect. Nothing frustrates me more than people who don't keep their word. People who make promises they have no intention of honoring or flake on commitments, throwing my plans into chaos.

October 9

I spoke with the attorney on Oahu about my wicked ex-stepmother. I walked away from my castle in 2014, but some small part of me still thought I could salvage something. The call was very enlightening on many levels. He said they tried to get the squatters out and resolve the issue so she could sell it. He said it would cost $20,000-40,000 to get them out with off-duty sheriffs from Oahu and Maui as there were not enough on the Big Island. They were waiting for it to go up for auction for back taxes. Today, the back taxes were $32,000. When I lived there, I paid the taxes diligently when they were due.

October 11

While scanning all my documents for *When We Wrote Letters*, I came across a letter from my cousin Lori, who spelled my name Sherry. Hey, we were young. When all this garbage went down, she told me cousin was a bully and pushed her around. I was noncommittal. Not that I didn't believe her; I just didn't want to get in the middle of drama, and we stopped speaking. Cousin's wife insisted that he wasn't physical with anyone. Then she left me a voice-mail saying that he hit her. I'm not surprised. I saved the voicemail. I got a wild hair to call Lori and apologize. Thankfully she accepted and we spoke for about two hours and caught up.

November 16

I had this crazy idea to call Annie, an old friend from my tweens, to ask her to help me find out where my mother was by calling cousin. He didn't pick up, but they texted:

Annie: I left my number on your VM a couple of days ago. I'm an old friend of Francine's. I want to send her a card.

Cousin: Fran is not able to speak with you.

Annie: Can I mail her a card? Address please.

Cousin: No.

Annie: Why not?

Cousin: Call Lori or Sheri.

Annie: Sheri gave me your number.

Then she said to me, "Sorry, he's such an a**." Yeah, so am I.

One day, I got up and went to take the shepherds out for their jog. Max was on one side of the scooter, Jasmine was on the other, and Bruiser was in the basket in the middle. People laughed and honked as they drove by. We started around the block, and I saw something black out of the corner of my eye on my neighbor's lawn. It was the bottom half of Magic. Tearfully,

I carried his body to the house, then something made me take the dogs down to the little park around the corner and there I found his top half with his collar. Magic had either been eaten by a coyote or killed by a raccoon. I doubted a coyote would leave so much of him. A year ago, he had a urinary blockage, which is common in male cats who eat kibble. It cost me $1,500 for emergency surgery at four in the morning. After Magic got eaten by a coyote, my neighbor came over and offered to mow my lawn. A kind gesture of condolence.

I dog sit. There is an app for that. Typically, the pet parents want to meet you and see where they will be leaving their pups. It's called a "meet and greet." While I was fostering Max and Jasmine, the dog had to meet the shepherds to see if everybody could play nicely. Nine times out of ten, they did, but there was always one percent that a dog was not submissive to Max, and then I couldn't sit for them.

November 25

Every Wednesday and Thursday some church people came with food to feed homeless people on a street in Fullerton. We fed about 20 to 60 people each time. Today is Thanksgiving. I brought pies that the owner of Northgate Gonzalez market generously donated and rolls from Panera Bread. God is great. As long as you keep giving and giving, blessings multiply and you receive more. The people who brought the meals said they are God-loving, and they pray before meals, but truly what they exhibit is critical and judgmental behavior. I'm done with them and will not go back. I wanted to tell them what I thought, but I was proud that I did not. God is teaching me how to live aloha and what it is to love and be loving and loved in return. All I could do was purse my lips tightly and hold my tongue. In the olden days, I would've told them point-blank what I thought. No filter.

2022

A year ago, I tried to donate blood to the Red Cross, and they said, "No, thank you." My hemoglobin was too low—12.5 g/dL was the minimum, and I was nowhere near it. I went to a hematologist, and after many tests and visits, he declared I was anemia-free and that I brought my blood levels up to the proper place in a year. I tried to give again—they still didn't want it. I was only a point off.

After years of attending NPE (Natural Product Expo), especially during my time in Hawaii, it was officially the end of an era. I called to register, though I wasn't exactly eager. The pandemic was still simmering, my arthritic knee screamed with every step, and the thought of hobbling through convention halls felt more like torture than an opportunity.

I told JoJo I have to work on Saturday, and she said, "You mean you GET to work on Saturday?" And I replied, "You're correct!" Mindful and grateful. Two such important concepts.

For the past two days, God had been testing me. I hope I passed with flying colors. Bettina, my 90-year-old friend, had a crisis of confusion. She had been sleeping her life away. I suggested things that she could occupy her time with. Then she said, "I'm 99," and I said, "No, you're not, you're 90." Her house reeked like cat poop. I told her I would change the litter for her. She had no litter. I went and bought some. Her dishes were piled up in the sink with pots and pans full of old, moldy food. I told her I would run the dishwasher. The next day, she called me at 8 p.m. and said, "I'm hungry, I want breakfast." And I said, "OK, but it's 8 p.m., how about dinner?" She thought it was 8 a.m. That was kind of scary. I told her I would come on Sunday and help her get organized, shop, and make sure she had food. She said she didn't know how much money she had. That was horrible to hear. I called FDS and asked him to make time for her on Sunday to take down her Christmas decorations. And this is why I don't decorate. Never have, never will. Watching Bettina deteriorate was heartbreaking. She was such a sweetheart. She ended up passing away a few months later.

February 1

I had a strong feeling, intuition at its best. I called the shepherds' mama, Katie, last night. She told me there is scuttlebutt that Alan and the submarine he is on might be returning by the end of this month! Music to my ears! I will finally be able to get my life back, and be able to get this house ready to make the improvements I need to make.

Brother Jeff informed me that they found a mass on his colon, and I've been spinning ever since he told me. The surgery will happen on February 7, and he will be in the hospital for a few days. Afterward, he is not allowed to lift more than ten pounds for three months. When he had his colonoscopy, they took out three polyps, which is no big deal, been there, done that. They saw a mass, took a little chunk, and told him that it was malignant. He freaked out. I freaked out. Then they backtracked and said they made a mistake, and it was not malignant. It got me thinking about *my* colonoscopy, I haven't had one in ten years. I didn't want to go into a hospital until this #CovidCrap passed. And now I'm wondering if I need to revisit that. How can I be so depressed one minute and then flying high the next? Does that mean I'm manic depressive?

I watched the special of Lady Gaga and Tony Bennett, who has dementia, and I longed for my mama. She is on my mind daily.

I met another Lynn—this one rescued kittens, so I dubbed her Rescue Mama to distinguish her from the others in my life. At one time, she had 15 little fosters who all needed to be bottle-fed. I offered to help, and there were two little girls who she named Tatiana and Oksana. We stand with Ukraine. I adopted them. It was time; I knew Magic approved. I'm calling them Tati and Sana.

February 28

I never planned to grow old alone. Hell, I never planned to be alone at any stage of my life, yet here I am. When I see couples that have been married for over 20, 30, or 40 years, I get a little sad and envious. That was supposed to be me. What the hell happened?

JoJo's friend Linda used to come over to play cards, always accompanied by her three-pound red Chihuahua, Roxy. One day, Linda asked her,

"If something happens to me, will you take Roxy?" Without hesitation, JoJo agreed. Tragically, just a few months later, Linda passed away suddenly, leaving JoJo with little Roxy. Thankfully, Roxy has since settled in comfortably to her new furever home.

JoJo had a long history of caring for others, having fostered numerous children over the years—so many, in fact, that she was featured in the local newspaper. One of her foster children, Margie, spent 14 years in the Air Force and now lives in Washington state. Despite the distance, Margie remained dedicated to JoJo, visiting several times a year to lend a hand. She put up and took down holiday decorations, she assisted during Gummy's decline, and supported JoJo with her granddaughter. Margie continued to be a steadfast presence in JoJo's life.

On March 9, the shepherds finally returned to their family. I'd miss them, sure—but not the endless barking, or the clouds of fur floating through the air. Having them for the past year has been quite the experience, but it's time for a return to what was my life pre-shepherds.

March 30

I swim thirty to sixty minutes every day for exercise and to get my Zen. FDS usually invited me to come over for dinner after swimming. He lived about five minutes from the gym. Bruiser was with me 24/7. He sat at the side of the pool and watched me swim and no one cared, I guess because he was so small. I had a service animal leash for him and an Rx from my doctor, so there was not much they could say.

When we got to FDS's, I carried him from the car into the house. After Magic was killed, I protected this little monkey because he liked to cruise and explore. The family and I ate dinner, and it was about 8:30 p.m. by the time we finished. I usually feed Bruiser between 6 and 8 p.m. so it was past his dinnertime. I knew he was starving. I had given the boy some chicken scraps, which he gobbled up. There was a knock at the door. A neighbor had a box of food she wanted to donate to the homeless. Sweet, right? Without anyone noticing, Bruiser slipped out the door. Five minutes later, I called for him to get ready to go home, but he didn't come. We searched the entire house before I headed outside in a panic. Everyone knew he wasn't allowed out on his own after Magic got eaten.

After ten minutes of calling his name, when he didn't come, I tried not to get frantic and think of coyotes. Little by little, all the people in the house came out to search. Pablo found Bruiser. His little stomach was eaten out. I put him in my car sobbing and drove home. I put him in a box in the freezer. FDS came the next day to dig a hole. We buried him next to Magic. FDS told me he looked at his surveillance camera and saw two coyotes in front of the house across the street. I imagined Bruiser probably went right up to them to play, and they grabbed him. For two days, all I did was sob. I didn't eat, didn't go anywhere. It's now Friday night and I finally ate an avocado. I lost five pounds in two days.

April 4

When you have a dog with you 24/7, there is nothing you can look at that doesn't provoke memories of your animal. Sitting in my car, I looked over to the passenger seat, and Bruiser was not there. I took him everywhere. I looked at the pillows on my bed. He used to crawl under them when people shot off fireworks. Now, when I hear a big boom, I'm almost relieved he is not here. I knew Bruiser was in a better place. If I am asked one more time by the people at the gym: "Where is your little dog?" I will scream. I swear I needed a billboard that said: my dog is dead; don't ask.

I was buying frozen food online from the Farmer's Dog for him and called to stop the auto-delivery. When they asked why, I had to tell them the reason. I was surprised by flowers at my door the next day. I had taken a picture of Bruiser and shared it with Dr. J. I knew he was the only one I could send a picture of Bruiser to because he wouldn't freak out seeing him shredded without his little tummy. He said I had PTSD.

June 23

I keep thinking about how I'd like to call my Mom and share what was going on in my life with her. What is normal anyway?

I see people on social media posting about their shiny lives, their possessions, their bling, and the next thing you know, they have it stolen or somehow it disappears. Such a surprise.

June 28

Thinking constantly of Ray, my Mom, Bruiser, and Gummy, all now gone from my life, made me reflect on others I've loved and also lost.

Dolly and Allen came to mind. We were part of the same Mormon ward in the '90s, and they shared my love for Hawaii. Dolly faced numerous physical challenges that eventually took their toll. After she passed, I helped Allen organize a celebration of life for her at the church, a luau—her favorite. And mine. Soon after, Allen started dating a woman in the ward who had also lost her spouse. I guess love found them in their grief. I don't know where they are now, but I miss Allen as a friend.

Maggie: In the '80s, we worked at a gentlemen's club, dancing with old farts. We both needed to earn money and met there. We didn't tell anyone because I think we thought people would think we had sex with them. It wasn't so. We both got "real" jobs and an apartment in Hollywood and became roommates. We dated horrible men who did lots of cocaine. They would share their cocaine in hopes of getting laid, and miracle of miracles couldn't get it up after they snorted an excessive amount of the drug. It had no effect on us, so we were amused by their stupidity. No fix for stupid. She went on to become a producer of one of my favorite cooking shows. She had a bad heart. She died in a "one car" accident, which I can only imagine was caused by her heart.

Kathy was my webmistress in the early 2000s and built the CastleInHawaii.com site. She passed, and I think of her often. She died despite her best efforts to be healthy. I still have a health book that she assembled in 2013 and emailed me. Topics included nerve food tea, lung purge, liver cleanse, kidney cleanse, and more archaic topics such as castor oil packs. Right now, I'm doing things regarding my diet and the way I live even more extreme after learning about best practices regarding Alzheimer's. Including sleep hygiene.

Allie was my sister-in-law, and we used to joke that it was a tie as to who got more screwed when we separated from J and his brother, her husband. He made a fortune in real estate and left her high and dry. Gee, no surprise there. I could write volumes about how he screwed not only J and our company but also one of our salespeople. I blamed myself for suggesting we all work together despite him being a competitor. In the end, Allie's behavior started feeling almost teenage—she stopped talking to me directly and would only communicate by text. No thanks. Eventually, she disappeared from my life altogether, never to return, and I miss her.

Allen has been my friend since the '70s. He is the one who saved my life by rescuing me from abuser #1, my first ex. I even contemplated moving to Florida to be with him. But he had an aversion to owning an animal. That was not an option in my reality. He's not dead, but I miss him in my life.

My self-worth has been tied to my income. Or lack thereof. Today is no different than it was in 1990. Why can't I just enjoy my life and be in the moment? I have another question for myself. Self? Why can't you just stop drinking alcohol? Even though it's not much, perhaps just a glass of red wine in the evening, it's impossible for me to just NOT drink. I hate that about myself. Hear that, self?

I'm adapting PP's memoir into a screenplay. This is probably the most anxiety-producing project I have ever worked on because it is PP's. I would never do anything to jeopardize our friendship. What if she hates it? Producer Jeff said, "She's not gonna hate it. She will love it." We decided to work on it together. He's up in Seattle. I'm down here in SoCal. We collaborated well.

Mega Millions jackpot hit $600 million jackpot, and I bought a ticket. I found a penny heads up, so I picked it up, and all day, I'm supposed to have good luck. I think I'll buy another ticket or two for the next drawing. It's ridiculous because I have not won even a dollar back on all the freaking tickets that I bought.

July 29

I wanted to earn passive income and learned about an opportunity to have a business coach. It was a company that had a course that taught you how to make a course. I want to make a Catering MasterClass. I just have to spend $6,800 if I want them to teach me how to do it. Spoiler alert: I paid them; I got taken. I got my money back because I'm just that kinda gal. I know others who didn't. I got an email saying those people filed a class action lawsuit against him.

August 5

Katy, Lydia's niece, sent me a text that began, "This is Lydia's niece ..." and at that moment, I didn't need to read any further—I knew what was coming. Cancer won. This would be horrible for her sister, who lived far away in the San Fernando Valley. Lydia lived alone (like me!) in South Orange County. They would have to deal with a house full of crap—dust, as I call it.

This got me thinking about my own stuff and my wish for my loved ones to come and choose what they want when I'm gone. I made a will, but there's always my lingering worry—did I forget to mention this item ... ? It's a delicate balance between holding on and letting go, even in preparation for after we're no longer here.

August 10

I stopped drinking alcohol. It was at PP's book launch. She had it at a venue in DTLA. She is my idol, my role model, my mentor, and my benefactress. I'm not sure how I got so lucky, but I never take it or her for granted. The event was so amazing! Over the top, and I wouldn't expect anything else. You entered the reception area to the sight of a champagne fountain sparkling in the center, while impeccably dressed waitstaff glided through the crowd, tray-passing the most exquisite mini tacos paired with shots of tequila. It wouldn't surprise me if it was the most expensive tequila in the world—but I couldn't say for sure, as tequila and I parted ways long ago. Then when we sat down to the meal. Each course had a different bottle of wine, fine wine, not crappy wine. And I am so proud to say I didn't have one drop of alcohol, and I was amazed. Friends were also amazed.

September 16

The word "rumination" kept echoing in my mind—a relentless loop of dwelling on problems, their causes, and consequences. I found myself trapped in it, unable to escape the constant replay of thoughts about my Mom and what she was going through. It gnawed at me, dragging me deeper into a spiral of distress. No matter how hard I tried, I just couldn't seem to stop.

Then I saw Robin Roberts interviewing Michelle Obama. As Michelle read from her book, her words struck me—because I could have written them. Mine would be: I look in the mirror and see a monster, a wrinkled, hollow-eyed monster with dark circles under the eyes. And that monster is me. Why do I carry such a distorted, cruel self-image?

Last night, I woke up at 4 a.m. with sharp pain in my left lower back, right where I imagined the kidneys were. When I wake in the middle of the night, I usually listen to a sleep story or meditate, but sometimes I turn on the TV. Last night, I decided to watch TV, and wouldn't you know it? Colbert was talking about kidney stones. Intuition? If this pain turns out to be a stone, how weird would that be? At times like this, I just want my mama. It's so hard not having her around.

October 21

I donated my day to Producer Jeff because he has been pouring money down the drain renting a storage space. When he was moving to Seattle, he wanted to get a storage unit, so I told him to get one in the OC so I could help in case he needed anything out of it.

He got a storage unit in Van Nuys near where he lived. After paying them almost $200 a month for the last two years, I told him I would give him a day to go there and pack stuff so he could get rid of it. I needed help because there was no way I could carry and lift all those boxes of stuff alone.

He's a talented artist, a true Pisces. Mostly he wanted me to ship his beautiful works of art to him. He paid FDS to come with me, and we emptied the storage unit. We went to the UPS store where I have my PO box for them to package and ship his things to him.

Every Friday night, Char is live (Charvision). I listened and always wished her Shabbat Shalom. I tried calling from two phones in rapid succession, and I finally got through! I waited patiently. I wanted to ask her if Lydia was around. But there wasn't time to ask her before time ran out and the show ended.

As I read the myriad of letters from my mother and my dads, all they did was talk about how much they loved me. It's weird to me that I never felt love.

Sometimes, I feel depressed, and other times ecstatic, jubilant, and joyful. I don't know how to keep the latter and get rid of the former. I was watching Selena Gomez share about her mental health in hopes of helping people. That's what I want to do by sharing my craziness about what happened to me. It was so painful.

A dear friend of mine, who was also a caterer, passed away on October 31. We shared great memories over the years, and one of my favorites was the time we went to CaterSource in New Orleans. We met Chef Paul Prudhomme, indulged in amazing food, and soaked up every bit of knowledge we could.

I attended her funeral at Forest Lawn, and I was struck by how modern everything had become. The whole process was automated. You could leave a message or memory on her tribute page, and it kept you updated with the date of the viewing, end of service details, and more. Reading through the messages from her other friends, I learned things I never knew, even after being friends for over twenty years. For instance, I had no idea she played the accordion!

Brother Jeff called today to let me know something was wrong with his dog, Duke. After a visit to the vet, he called again to share the news that Duke had a heart murmur, and his stomach was swollen with fluid. The vet gave him several medications and sent them home, but Duke passed away not long after.

I am down to 125 pounds from clean eating. I haven't had a drop of alcohol since August 10, 2022. the day of PP's book launch. Do I miss it? Hell, yes! Am I glad I quit? Hell, yes! I love my brain too much to keep doing something harmful to it. The one thing that J gave me from our 25+ years together was that once you know something, then you're responsible for it, and that is one lesson I cannot forget every time it comes up in my life.

October 23, Mom's Birthday

Not being able to speak to Mom on her birthday felt like an unfillable void. It used to be a day we shared on our birthdays – hers or mine. Whether through a phone call or if possible, a visit. Now, the silence is deafening. It's not just the loss of the conversation. It's the loss of the ritual, the connection, the comfort of knowing that she was there, just a call away. Not hearing her voice, not sharing what was going on like we used to, leaves a hole, reminding me that no matter how much time passes, some losses never really heal.

Lydia's sister gave me the butterflies from Lydia's bedroom wall. It is a metal sculpture and is unique and exquisite. That was another thing we shared. Our love for butterflies, mermaids, Hawaii, eating healthy, taking supplements. I knew exactly where I would put it. There is a blank space on the front of the house between the two-bedroom windows. Every time I come home, I will see it and think about her. I know she is watching over me and watching out for me.

December 31

Lin came in from Chicago for New Year's. We went to a cryotherapy place. You get into a big tank, and they raise you so that your head sticks up over it, and then they flood the tank with nitrogen. There are levels of negative degrees, and I went in at the least cold, while Lin went in at the coldest. You wear socks, gloves, and a robe to begin. You then remove the robe but keep the socks and the gloves on. I had to dance to make it to three minutes.

I made a big, beautiful, healthy salad, and we stuffed our pie holes at about 3 p.m. because we couldn't go on without some nourishment. Cryo burns calories and makes you hungry. After that, we went into an infrared sauna at 140° for 45 minutes. Then we went to her hotel and soaked in the jacuzzi. A perfect day.

PP's hubby tested positive for Covid, so I went with my bag full of potions and supplements and everything I knew of to get him better in a hurry. I bought a head of garlic and roasted it; I gave them a green smoothie with turmeric in it and went to buy wheatgrass juice. I dosed them both with my concoction of oregano, rosemary, olive leaf, maitake mushroom homeopathic drops, and elderberry extract.

Nowadays, I meditate daily. Does that mean I am a Buddhist? Perhaps I am Jewish, born again, Kabbalist, Buddhist. I believe in covering my bases. People say I have had an interesting life. Where's my shrug emoji? It was just a life and a lifetime ago. I guess since I'm from a "showbiz" family, that's fascinating to some.

PET PEEVES—I HAVE A FEW (Doesn't Everyone?)

1. Stupid Drivers: There's no fix for stupid drivers who don't pay attention to the road or blast music so loudly they can't hear what's happening around them. The same goes for people walking with earbuds in, oblivious to their surroundings, watching their device instead of paying attention to where they are going.

2. Traffic Signal Etiquette: People who stop far from the sensor at the crosswalk and wonder why the light won't change.

3. Extreme Mask-Wearing: People wearing masks alone in their cars or

combining mask-wearing with un-healthy habits, like smoking or eating fast food.

4. Conspiracy Theorists: Not a fan of people who spread disinformation and conspiracy theories as if it's gospel truth.

5. Social Media insanity and doom scrolling: People who share every moment of their shiny lives or post every mundane detail, down to what color toilet paper they used. (Taken to the extreme, kidding but you get the point…?). Or post pics of their bling and wonder why they get it stolen. Or wish their spouse a Happy Birthday or Anniversary on social. Why don't they just pick up the phone? And why do people feel compelled to give an opinion and advice about something whether they were asked to or not.

6. Tagging Property: People who feel entitled to deface property with graffiti or "tags." The people who do it call it art, isn't that called vandalism?

7. "Gentle Leaders": I'm an old-school dog trainer: a collar and a choke chain worked for years. If it ain't broke, why fix it.

8. Halloween Madness: Let's send kids out to trick or treat, then warn them about razors and drugs in their candy. Sounds like a great idea—not.

9. Medical (drug) Commercials: It seems like a constant barrage. It used to be illegal, I believe. Thank goodness for DVR to fast-forward through them.

10. Thankless drivers: I let someone go ahead of me, and they don't even nod or smile. Is basic courtesy really that hard? A nod, acknowledgement, a wave?

11. Health Posts/Disclosures: Why do people feel the need to post their medical challenges on social media for the world to see? HIPAA was created to protect our sensitive health information and ensure our privacy, yet many are quick to disclose it without a second thought.

12. Instant Honkers: People who honk the second the light turns green. Seriously?

13. Obligatory gift giving because it is expected. For example, giving gifts because it's Christmas. I prefer giving gifts when it feels right, not because I'm supposed to.

14. Lottery Obsession: My guilty pleasure—throwing money at the lottery because you have to "be in it to win it", right? I can't resist even though I'm aware of how great the odds are.

15. Animal tail docking and ear cropping and declawing cats: In my opinion? It's cruel and unnecessary.

THINGS I'VE LEARNED AND KNOW FOR SURE:

1. If you think you can or you think you can't—YOU'RE RIGHT! *(If you think you can: how? I say: focus, focus, focus)*

2. Hindsight is twenty-twenty.

3. What you think of me is none of my business.

4. Bend like a willow, or snap like an oak.

5. No expectations, no disappointments.

6. Everybody lies. And there are three sides to every story, yours mine and the truth.

7. Knowledge is power. I often wonder if I can share every bit of wisdom in my

brain to help others. Probably not, but I'll try.

8. Don't delete texts. Keeping the history helps you recall conversations later.

9. Spend that extra dollar on the cloud for your phone contacts—why lose data when you don't have to?

10. Use the right tool for the job. You wouldn't dig a grave with a teaspoon. Likewise, don't use your teeth for anything but eating—especially if you have caps—and avoid using your fingernails as tools if you like keeping them long and lovely.

My thoughts on grief?

I must embrace the grief that comes from all the unspoken love I never got to share with my Mom. My cousin stole the chance for me to be there with her and for her at the end, but the grief that remains is now my connection to her. Forget the inheritance (the dust)—this pain is what's left. Though heavy, it carries the unexpressed love and the lessons I was denied, making it a precious link to her memory.

I heard so many profound things on Anderson Cooper's podcast (thank you for this Anderson!), but these in particular resonated with me deeply:

> Everyone has gone through or will go through grief.

> Grief is love with nowhere to go. It lingers as a reminder of what was, and the absence that now fills the space.

> Grief is the enormity of the room whose door has quietly shut leaving only silence.

> Grief is not a bad thing, it's a reaction to a bad thing.

Yes yes yes and yes. It seems grief rewires you and sneaks into moments you don't expect. You're never the same afterward. And maybe that's okay.

Epilogue

I heard that cousin sold the New York apartment
and moved with his wife into my Mom's house.
I could only imagine that they used her money
to remodel it. Then I learned the house was up
for sale. Whether he had her change her will
or estate documents doesn't even matter. If that
were true, people without capacity aren't allowed
to sign anything—it's against the law. Unless
you've got boatloads of money, taking someone

to court for justice is a waste of time. In the end, it's all just dust. You can't take it with you.

One of cousin's sons texted me a picture of an infant: "Hey. I hope all is well with you. I wanted to let you know my wife just gave birth to my son. The other thing, a sad one, is that I heard through the grapevine that your mom passed away recently. I just wanted to send my condolences. I'm very sorry for you, and I know they can be very tough. I'm busy right now but can call you tomorrow."

Recently? I got Mama's death certificate. She died on May 20, 2023, at her house. It says on her death certificate cousin had her cremated. **She wanted to be buried next to Don.** Am I shouting? How do I really feel? It was probably cheaper. What I'd like to know is: where are her ashes???

They listed the cause of death as hypertensive cardiovascular disease. Why does it matter? If I decided to take him to court, he could say she signed everything over to him and wasn't incapacitated. Plus "if" I took him to court, Julie, her caregiver, said SHE SAW him have her sign a document.

What kind of person would keep a woman in her 60s away from her mother, who was in her late 80s? I try to be the bigger person and pray for him. I even practice loving-kindness meditations for him: *"May you be safe, may you be healthy, may you be happy, and may you live with ease."* But let's be real—he's a sick individual—and a criminal to boot. Yes, that's a judgment call, but one based on his actions.

For some people, money and possessions are all that matters. I still ask why, why, why, why? You can't take it with you, and it serves no purpose. Yes, I guess life can be more comfortable with all those things, but I'd rather give to others, as Kabbalah teaches. That's just me. "Don't tell Sheri." What a guy. And in the end, what did he really win?

Acknowledgments

To my readers—thank you for your patience, and for joining me on this journey. Your support means everything. To the kind and gracious Susie Singer Carter, who took time out of her busy life to give feedback on some pages, even when she didn't really have time. Although it's too late for her mama, may her documentary save many lives!

Huge mahalo to my dear friend and neighbor, Lyn, my beta editor, for holding my feet to the fire and encouraging me to keep going, even when I wanted to give up. Your guidance and belief in this project were invaluable. And to one of my oldest and best friends since eighth grade-Sarah, Sea, my love. You know why!

My beloved PP, thank you for standing by me and offering unwavering support after my return from Hawaii losing everything. You are a true source of strength in my life.

Brother Jeff (my Hānai brother) and Producer Jeff—what can I say? Without you, I wouldn't want to be here, let alone write. You are truly my dearest friends, and I'm endlessly grateful for your friendship and encouragement.

A special thank you to my editor, Mary Rembert, for your insightful suggestions and for believing in my voice and my story. Your feedback pushed me to dig deeper and craft something authentic.

To Dr. J for immortalizing my boy on the front of his book PaleoPet.guide and being my friend for over thirty years.

To my friends (especially my Mexican ohanas), both past and present, who shaped me and my story. FDS and his HUGE Family, JoJo and her HUGE family, Cecilia and her HUGE family. To my friend Lynn, whose heart for rescuing is bigger than anyone could imagine. She tirelessly dedicates herself to rescuing animals in need. And to my loving and kind neighbors.

And finally, to all the friends and mentors who have supported me, read the "arc" (advanced reader copy), listened, and reminded me to stay true to myself—you know who you are. I appreciate you deeply.

Thank you all for being part of this journey and for holding space for my story.

About the Author

Sheri Smith considers herself fortunate to have discovered lifelong passions: catering, events, and creative writing. Her work journey began at age seven, starring on Broadway and appearing in the longest-running M&M commercial in the 60s. In the 70s, Sheri enlisted in the Navy, aspiring to become an EMT, but societal limitations shifted her back to the entertainment industry.

In '90, she bought a catering company (GourmetCatering.com), serving prestigious clients across Southern California. After 9/11, she moved to the Big Island of Hawaii, where she built a castle-themed vacation rental that gained media attention. She traveled back and forth to the mainland for events.

Today, Sheri focuses on ChocolateFountain SoCal.com because it never gets old and (food and beverage) catering ranging from intimate weddings to large corporate events while continuing to explore new creative endeavors. She stays active with daily swimming, gym workouts, and pupsitting. When not catering, Sheri continues to write and explore new creative endeavors.

For updates and future releases: Buy Now or Follow the Author

SheriSmithAuthor.com

www.ingramcontent.com/pod-product-compliance
Lightning Source LLC
Chambersburg PA
CBHW042137140626
46547CB00038B/724